AF841916

TransOral Robotic Surgery for Obstructive Sleep Apnea

Claudio Vicini • Paul T. Hoff
Filippo Montevecchi
Editors

TransOral Robotic Surgery for Obstructive Sleep Apnea

A Practical Guide to Surgical Approach and Patient Management

Springer

Editors
Claudio Vicini
Head and Neck Department - ENT & Oral Surgery Unit - G.B. Morgagni - L. Pierantoni Hospital
Forlì – Infermi Hospital
Faenza - ASL of Romagna, Italy

Filippo Montevecchi
Head and Neck Department - ENT & Oral Surgery Unit - G.B. Morgagni - L. Pierantoni Hospital
Forlì – Infermi Hospital
Faenza - ASL of Romagna, Italy

Paul T. Hoff
Department of Otolaryngology - Head and Neck Surgery Ann Arbor
University of Michigan Health System
Michigan, USA

ISBN 978-3-319-34038-8 ISBN 978-3-319-34040-1 (eBook)
DOI 10.1007/978-3-319-34040-1

Library of Congress Control Number: 2016950727

© Springer International Publishing Switzerland 2016
This work is subject to copyright. All rights are reserved by the Publisher, whether the whole or part of the material is concerned, specifically the rights of translation, reprinting, reuse of illustrations, recitation, broadcasting, reproduction on microfilms or in any other physical way, and transmission or information storage and retrieval, electronic adaptation, computer software, or by similar or dissimilar methodology now known or hereafter developed.
The use of general descriptive names, registered names, trademarks, service marks, etc. in this publication does not imply, even in the absence of a specific statement, that such names are exempt from the relevant protective laws and regulations and therefore free for general use.
The publisher, the authors and the editors are safe to assume that the advice and information in this book are believed to be true and accurate at the date of publication. Neither the publisher nor the authors or the editors give a warranty, express or implied, with respect to the material contained herein or for any errors or omissions that may have been made.

Printed on acid-free paper

This Springer imprint is published by Springer Nature
The registered company is Springer International Publishing AG Switzerland

Foreword

TransOral Robotic Surgery (TORS) for Obstructive Sleep Apnea (OSA) is further proof of the significant applications and role of robotic surgery in the head and neck surgery and otolaryngology. In less than 10 years TORS for OSA has spread all around the world, and the diffusion of this technique may be traced through the increasing number of published papers in the literature. While the initial focus of TORS in the USA was on its application for oropharyngeal cancer, however the potential and implication for a substantial role in the surgical treatment of OSA was clear. First thoughts on the potential of TORS for OSA arose incidentally in the early phases of the first human clinical trials for TORS at Penn. Fortuitously, a patient enrolled in the trial and undergoing TORS tongue base resection to rule out tumor or lymphoma enlightened us that she was sleeping much better after her TORS procedure. It was then that planning to develop a strategy to test TORS for OSA was initiated and then a relationship with Claudio Vicini was formed. It was in March of 2008 that Claudio Vicini and Filippo Montevecchi visited the University of Pennsylvania to learn how to develop a TORS program in Italy. They spent time with us, learning our approach, and returned home to Italy to develop their premiere program in TORS. The first TORS tongue base reduction for OSA was carried out in May 2008 in Forlì by Vicini and Montevecchi. The surgery was planned after more than 1 year of training in Italy, France (IRCAD, Strasbourg), and the USA (Philadelphia, PA). This book is the first on TORS written expressly for treating sleep apnea patients affected by a hypertrophy of the tongue base.

In 2009 the Food and Drug Administration (FDA) approved the use of TORS for upper airway T1 and T2 cancers as well as "benign disease" of the pharynx. The sleep apnea experience in the USA grew from a small cohort of surgeons training alongside their head and neck oncology colleagues. The introduction of TORS coincided with the popularization of Drug Induced Sedated Endoscopy (DISE) in the USA. TORS in the USA is now largely performed by surgeons who routinely incorporate DISE as part of their preoperative assessment. The experience with TORS between 2010 and 2014 led to the FDA approval (September 2014) of TORS for "removal of benign tissue from the base of tongue." No specification about the indication for tongue base benign tissue removal was offered. Prospective trials to assess both safety and efficacy are currently under way.

TORS for OSA may now be considered a routine surgical procedure in many otolaryngology and head and neck surgery practices throughout the world, and we are seeing a steep rise in the number of new cases being performed annually. The implications of this increasing activity are many and may be complex, as every institution faces its own individual challenges in establishing a successful TORS sleep program. The aim of this book is to provide an important set of information about TORS for OSA and stimulate those to develop their own robotic skill sets and apply them to treat this devastating and surgically challenging disease.

Bert W. O'Malley Jr.
Gabriel Tucker Professor and Chairman
Department of Otorhinolaryngology - Head and Neck Surgery
Associate Vice President,
Director Physician Network Development
The University of Pennsylvania Health System,
Philadelphia, PA, USA

Gregory S. Weinstein
Professor and Vice Chair
Director, Division of Head and Neck Surgery Co-Director,
The Center for Head and Neck Cancer Department of
Otorhinolaryngology - Head and Neck Surgery
The University of Pennsylvania Health System
Philadelphia, PA, USA
March 2016

Preface

πάντα ῥεῖ (everything flows)

Hērákleitos, Ephésios; c. 535–c. 475 BCE

Why one more robotic book focused on a single application? And why about sleep apnea? Does this new book justify the effort? Is this work a significant contribution to this emerging field? Last but not least, is there an audience for this body of work? From our perspective on the front line of sleep surgery research, all the questions deserve an affirmative answer.

In the worldwide literature there are many excellent books dealing with TORS and most of them include a chapter about OSA, but it's just a chapter inside a book mostly dedicated to head and neck cancer surgery; many important details regarding basic topics in the OSA application are described in a brief and cursory way. Sleep apnea is among the most prevalent diseases in the world and its incidence has increased dramatically over the last two decades.

CPAP has long been considered the "Gold Standard" therapy for OSA; however it is not accepted or is discontinued by a significant number of subjects, opening the door for alternative options, including surgery. Recent progress in drug-induced sleep endoscopy has demonstrated a central role of tongue base obstruction in at least one third of the moderate to severe cases; tongue base obstruction is the ideal target for robotic surgery.

Many of the traditional surgical options for tongue base proved to be effective but did not gain widespread acceptance due to significant morbidity. It is probably for all the above listed considerations that in the last decade TORS for OSA, the most recent option in tongue base reduction, has quickly become the most published single procedure for managing tongue base obstruction in sleep apnea. For the same reason, many centers around the world have now introduced TORS for OSA within their established head and neck oncology programs. With the increasing demand to apply TORS to OSA, many of the authors of this book have shared their experiences in innumerable meetings, courses, proctoring, and case observations. The aim of this book has been to put together a comprehensive evaluation and treatment paradigm for surgeons treating patients with OSA. The surgical treatment will focus on preoperative DISE as well as a multilevel surgical treatment plan with a special focus on TORS. TORS specific topics include how to optimize surgery and how to deal with the possible complications and failures.

Finally, this book is written by surgeons for surgeons and reflects different solutions adopted in different countries according to the different health care management rules, experiences, backgrounds, economic situation, surgeons, and patients culture. Each chapter is written by a team of surgeons representing perspectives from no less than two different countries. We have tried to offer the reader a wide perspective in order to allow the information to fit individual surgeons and programs circumstances. The book is unique in offering a complete body of detailed information encompassing TORS for OSA: patient selection, preoperative work up, anesthesia, pre- and postoperative management, multilevel surgery including TORS, complication prevention and management, and approaches to surgical failures. A special feature is the essential description of the sleep medicine and sleep surgery background, required for correct patient selection. Sleep medicine and sleep surgery expertise is usually not common among TORS Surgeons, most of whom come from a head and neck oncology background. The final chapters may help surgeons from different geographic areas to recognize the specific challenges of running a dedicated TORS program for OSA in their own countries.

Last but not least we would like to thank all the people who have made this effort possible. First of all our institutions, which gave us the technological and human resources that allowed us to develop a pioneering role in the development of TORS for OSA. A special mention for the Cassa dei Risparmi Foundation of Forlì which was crucial in supporting the robotic program at our institution. Then our co-workers (ENT partners, residents, fellows, etc.) who shared with us the daily effort to improve our techniques and patient care. A special mention to all our colleagues outside of otolaryngology (sleep doctors, anesthesiologists, etc.) and to our nursing staff, for their very supportive cooperation. We cannot overestimate the role of our common mentors, Greg Weinstein and Bert O'Malley, who gave us the fundamentals and inspirations to pioneer the use of the robotic approach in sleep surgery.

This very rewarding, but time-consuming job would not have been possible without the love and warm support of our families. Many thanks to all of them!

Forlì, Italy — Claudio Vicini
Forlì, Italy — Filippo Montevecchi
Ann Arbor, MI, USA — Paul Theodore Hoff

Contents

1 **Introduction** ... 1
Claudio Vicini, Filippo Montevecchi, and Paul T. Hoff

Part I Patient Work-Up

2 **Tongue Pathophysiology in OSAS Patients: A Surgically Oriented Perspective** ... 7
Filippo Montevecchi, Claudio Vicini, Matteo Costantini, Riccardo Gobbi, Elisabetta Firinu, Ottavio Piccin, and Giovanni Sorrenti

3 **History-Taking and Clinical Examination** ... 13
Claudio Vicini, Filippo Montevecchi, Paul Hoff, Claudia Zanotti, Tod Huntley, and Yassin Bahgat

4 **Sleep Studies** ... 21
Brian W. Rotenberg, Marcello Bosi, Sabrina Frassineti, and Venerino Poletti

5 **Imaging** ... 33
Andrea De Vito, Pier Carlo Frasconi, Oscar Bazzocchi, and Giulia Tenti

6 **Drug-Induced Sedation Endoscopy (DISE)** ... 41
Aldo Campanini, Bhik Kotecha, and Erica R. Thaler

7 **Patient Selection** ... 51
Tiffany Ann Glazer, Paul T. Hoff, Matthew E. Spector, Claudio Vicini, Filippo Montevecchi, Neil S. Tolley, and Asit Arora

Part II Surgery

8 **Transoral Robotic Surgery as Single Level Surgery for Treatment of Obstructive Sleep Apnea** ... 63
Ho-Sheng Lin

9 **TORS in a Multilevel Procedure** ... 71
Ahmed Bahgat, Ehsan Hendawy, Kenny P. Pang, and Claudio Vicini

10 **Alternative Procedures** ... 77
Mohamed Eesa, Ahmed Bahgat, and Ehsan Hendawy

11 **Robotic Setting** ... 83
Mark A. D'Agostino, Gregory A. Grillone, and Federico Faedi

12 **Surgical Anatomy in Transoral Robotic Procedure: Basic Fundamentals** ... 91
Iacopo Dallan, Lodovica Cristofani-Mencacci, Giovanni D'Agostino, Ermelinda Zeccardo, and Hesham Negm

13 **Transoral Robotic Surgery for Obstructive Sleep Apnea Syndrome: An Anesthetist's Point of View** ... 109
Ruggero Massimo Corso, Davide Cattano, and Nabil Abdelhamid Shallik

14 **Technique: How We Do It** ... 121
Claudio Vicini, Filippo Montevecchi, and J. Scott Magnuson

Part III Post-Operative Concerns

15 **Postoperative Management of Transoral Robotic Surgery for Obstructive Sleep Apnea** ... 139
Chiara Marchi and Julia A. Crawford

16 **Expected Outcomes** ... 143
Claudio Vicini, Filippo Montevecchi, Aldo Campanini, Iacopo Dallan, Paul T. Hoff, Matthew E. Spector, Erica R. Thaler, Jeffrey Ahn, Peter M. Baptista, Marc Remacle, Georges Lawson, Marco Benazzo, and Pietro Canzi

17 **Complication Management** ... 151
Filippo Montevecchi, Saleh Ali AlGhamdi, and Chiara Bellini

18 **Short- and Long-Term Dysphagia** ... 159
Mohamed Eesa and Giuseppe Meccariello

19 **Failures Management** ... 167
Claudio Vicini, Claudia Zanotti, L. B. L. Benoist, Gianluca Giorgio Marrano, and Nico de Vries

Part IV TORS for OSAS in Geographic Perspective: How to Run a Program in Different Countries

20 **The North American Experience** ... 175
Paul T. Hoff, Robson Capasso, and Umamaheswar Duvvuri

21 The South American Experience 183
Eric R. Thuler, Fábio A.W. Rabelo, and Fabiana C.P. Valera

22 The European Experience 187
Asit Arora, Bhik Kotecha, Tom Vauterin, Guillermo Plaza, Christian Güldner, and Jochen A. Werner

23 The Middle East Experience 197
Medhat Shams and Hayam Altaweel

24 The Far Eastern Asian Experience 203
Song Tar Toh and Vikas Agrawal

25 The Australian Experience 209
Suren Krishnan and Julia A. Crawford

Part V Research and Future Perspectives

26 Research and Future Perspectives 215
Claudio Vicini, Filippo Montevecchi, Paul T. Hoff, Asit Arora, and E. Vetri

Index 225

Contributors

Vikas Agrawal, MS, FCPS, DORL Department of ENT, Speciality ENT Hospital, Mumbai, India

Jeffrey M. Ahn, MD Department of Otolaryngology – Head and Neck Surgery, Columbia University Medical Center, New York, NY, USA

Saleh Ali AlGhamdi, MD ENT Department, King Fahd Armed Forces Hospital, Jeddah, Kingdom of Saudi Arabia

Hayam Altaweel, FACH, ARZT Department of Otolaryngology – Head and Neck Surgery, Hamad Medical Corporation, Doha, Qatar

Asit Arora, DIC, FRCS Department of Otorhinolaryngology and Head & Neck Surgery, St. Mary's Hospital, Imperial College Healthcare NHS Trust, London, UK

Ahmed Bahgat, MD, MSc, EBE Department of Otorhinolaryngology—Head & Neck Surgery, Alexandria University, Alexandria, Egypt

Yassin Bahgat, MD, MSc, EBE Department of Otorhinolaryngology—Head & Neck Surgery, Alexandria University, Alexandria, Egypt

Peter M. Baptista, MD, PhD Department of ORL, Clinica Universidad de Navarra, Pamplona, Spain

Oscar Bazzocchi, MD Radiology Unit, G.B. Morgagni—L. Pierantoni Hospital, Forlì, Italy

Chiara Bellini, MD Head and Neck Department—ENT & Oral Surgery Unit, G.B. Morgagni—L. Pierantoni Hospital, ASL of Romagna, Forlì, Italy

Infermi Hospital, ASL of Romagna, Faenza, Italy

Marco Benazzo, MD, PhD Department of Otolaryngology, IRCCS Policlinico San Matteo, University of Pavia, Pavia, Italy

L.B.L. Benoist, MD Department of Otolaryngology, OLVG Location West, Amsterdam, The Netherlands

Marcello Bosi, MD Pulmonary Operative Unit, Department of Thoracic Diseases, G.B. Morgagni–L. Pierantoni Hospital, Forlì, Italy

Aldo Campanini, MD Head and Neck Department—ENT & Oral, Surgery Unit G.B. Morgagni—L. Pierantoni Hospital, ASL of Romagna, Forlì, Italy

Infermi Hospital, ASL of Romagna, Faenza, Italy

Pietro Canzi, MD Department of Otolaryngology, IRCCS Policlinico San Matteo, University of Pavia, Pavia, Italy

Robson Capasso, MD Department of Otolaryngology – Head and Neck Surgery, Sleep Surgery Division, Stanford University Medical Center, Stanford, CA, USA

Davide Cattano, MD, PhD UTH Medical School at Houston, Houston, TX, USA

Ruggero Massimo Corso, MD Emergency Department, Anesthesia and Intensive Care Section, G.B. Morgagni—L. Pierantoni Hospital, Forlì, Italy

Matteo Costantini, MD Department of Pathology, Head and Neck Department, Transfusion and Laboratory Medicine, GB Morgagni – L Pierantoni Hospital, Forlì, Italy

Julia A. Crawford, BSc, MBBS, FRACS Department of Otolaryngology, Head and Neck Surgery, St Vincent's Hospital, Darlinghurst, NSW, Australia

Giovanni D'Agostino Head and Neck Department—ENT & Oral Surgery Unit, G.B. Morgagni—L. Pierantoni Hospital, ASL of Romagna, Forlì, Italy; Infermi Hospital, ASL of Romagna, Faenza, Italy

Mark A. D'Agostino, M.D., F.A.C.S. Department of Otolaryngology – Head & Neck Surgery, Middlesex Hospital, Middletown, CT, USA

Southern New England Ear, Nose and Throat Group, New Haven, CT, USA

Iacopo Dallan, MD First ENT Unit, Azienda Ospedaliero-Universitaria Pisana, Pisa, Italy

Head and Neck Surgery & Forensic Dissection Research Center (HNS & FDRC), Department of Biotechnology and Life Sciences (DBSV), University of Insubria, Varese, Italy

Nico de Vries, MD, PhD Department of Otolaryngology, OLVG Location West, Amsterdam, The Netherlands

Department of Otolaryngology, University of Antwerp, Antwerp, Belgium

Andrea De Vito, MD, PhD Head and Neck Department—ENT & Oral, Surgery Unit G.B. Morgagni—L. Pierantoni Hospital, Forli - Infermi Hospital, Faenza - ASL of Romagna, Italy

Umamaheswar Duvvuri, MD, PhD Department of Otolaryngology, University of Pittsburgh, Pittsburgh, PA, USA

Mohamed Eesa, M.D., M.Sc., E.B.E. Department of Otolaryngology, Head–Neck Surgery, University of Zagazig, Zagazig, Egypt

Federico Faedi, MS, Engineering Head and Neck Department—ENT & Oral Surgery Unit, G.B. Morgagni—L. Pierantoni Hospital, Forli - Infermi Hospital, Faenza - ASL of Romagna, Italy

Elisabetta Firinu, MD Head and Neck Department—ENT & Oral Surgery Unit, G.B. Morgagni—L. Pierantoni Hospital, Forli - Infermi Hospital, Faenza - ASL of Romagna, Italy

Pier Carlo Frasconi, MD Head and Neck Department—ENT & Oral Surgery Unit G.B. Morgagni—L. Pierantoni Hospital, Forli – Infermi Hospital, Faenza – ASL of Romagna, Italy

Sabrina Frassineti, MD Head and Neck Department—ENT & Oral Surgery Unit, G.B. Morgagni–L. Pierantoni Hospital, ASL of Romagna, Forlì, Italy

Infermi Hospital, ASL of Romagna, Faenza, Italy

Tiffany Ann Glazer, MD Department of Otolaryngology – Head and Neck Surgery, University of Michigan Health System, Ann Arbor, MI, USA

Riccardo Gobbi, MD Head and Neck Department—ENT & Oral Surgery Unit, G.B. Morgagni—L. Pierantoni Hospital, Forli - Infermi Hospital, Faenza - ASL of Romagna, Italy

Gregory A. Grillone, MD, FACS Department of Otolaryngology, Boston University Medical Center, Boston, MA, USA

Christian Güldner, MD, PhD University Hospital of Essen, Essen, Germany

Ehsan Hendawy, M.D., M.Sc., E.B.E Department of Otolaryngology, Head–Neck Surgery, University of Zagazig, Zagazig, Egypt

Paul T. Hoff, MS, MD Department of Otolaryngology – Head and Neck Surgery, University of Michigan Health System, Ann Arbor, MI, USA

Tod Huntley, MD, FACS CENTA: Center for Ear Nose Throat & Allergy, Carmel, IN, USA

Bhik Kotecha, MBBCh, MPhil, FRCS Royal National Throat, Nose & Ear Hospital, London, UK

Suren Krishnan, MBBS, FRACS Department of Otolaryngology, Head and Neck Surgery, Royal Adelaide Hospital, Adelaide, SA, Australia

Georges Lawson, MD Department of ORL-Head & Neck Surgery, Louvain University Hospital of Mont Godinne, Yvoir, Belgium

Ho-Sheng Lin, MD Department of Otolaryngology—Head & Neck Surgery, Wayne State University, Detroit, MI, USA

Department of Surgery, John D Dingell VA Medical Center, Detroit, MI, USA

J. Scott Magnuson, MD Department of Head and Neck Surgery, Florida Hospital Celebration Health, Celebration, FL, USA

Chiara Marchi, MD Head and Neck Department—ENT & Oral Surgery Unit, G.B. Morgagni—L. Pierantoni Hospital, ASL of Romagna, Forlì, Italy

Infermi Hospital, ASL of Romagna, Faenza, Italy

Gianluca Giorgio Marrano, MD Head and Neck Department—ENT & Oral Surgery Unit, G.B. Morgagni—L. Pierantoni Hospital, ASL of Romagna, Forlì, Italy

Infermi Hospital, ASL of Romagna, Faenza, Italy

Giuseppe Meccariello, MD Head and Neck Department—ENT & Oral Surgery Unit, G.B. Morgagni—L. Pierantoni Hospital, ASL of Romagna, Forlì, Italy

Infermi Hospital, ASL of Romagna, Faenza, Italy

Lodovica Cristofani-Mencacci, MD First ENT Unit, Azienda Ospedaliero-Universitaria Pisana, Pisa, Italy

Filippo Montevecchi, MD Head and Neck Department - ENT & Oral Surgery Unit - G.B. Morgagni - L. Pierantoni Hospital, Forlì – Infermi Hospital, Faenza - ASL of Romagna, Italy

Hesham Negm, MB BCh, MSc, MD Department of Otorhinolaryngology, Faculty of Medicine, Cairo University, Cairo, Egypt

Kenny Peter Pang, MBBS, MRCS, FRCS Department of Otolaryngology, Asia Sleep Centre, Paragon Medical, Singapore, Singapore

Ottavio Piccin, MD, MSc Otolaryngoloy and Audiology Unit, Head and Neck Surgery, Sant'Orsola-Malpighi Hospital, Bologna University, Bologna, Italy

Guillermo Plaza, MD, PhD Hospital Universitario de Fuenlabrada and Hospital Sanitas La Zarzuela, Fuenlabrada, Spain

Venerino Poletti, MD Pulmonary Operative Unit, Department of Thoracic Diseases, G.B. Morgagni–L. Pierantoni Hospital, Forlì, Italy

Department of Respiratory Diseases & Allergology, Aarhus University Hospital, Aarhus, Denmark

Fábio A.W. Rabelo, MD, PhD Robotic Surgery Center at Oswaldo Cruz German Hospital, São Paulo, Brazil

Marc Remacle, MD, PhD Department of ORL-Head & Neck Surgery, Louvain University Hospital of Mont Godinne, Yvoir, Belgium

Brian W. Rotenberg, MD, MPH, FRCSC Department of Otolaryngology—Head & Neck Surgery, Western University, London, ON, Canada

Nabil Abdelhamid Shallik, MB, ChB, MSc, MD Anesthesia, ICU and Perioperative Medicine Department, Hamad Medical Corporation, Doha, Qatar

Department of Anesthesia, ICU and Perioperative Medicine, Hamad Medical Corporation, Qatar, Doha, Qatar

Medhat Shams, MD Department of Otolaryngology – Head and Neck Surgery, Hamad Medical Corporation, Rumailah Hospital, Doha, Qatar

Giovanni Sorrenti, MD Otolaryngoloy and Audiology Unit, Head and Neck Surgery, Sant'Orsola-Malpighi Hospital, Bologna University, Bologna, Italy

Matthew E. Spector, MD Department of Otolaryngology – Head and Neck Surgery, University of Michigan Health System, Ann Arbor, MI, USA

Giulia Tenti, MD Centro Chirurgico Toscano, Arezzo, Italy

Erica R. Thaler, MD, FACS Division of General Otolaryngology, Head and Neck Surgery, Department of Otolaryngology-Head and Neck Surgery, University of Pennsylvania School of Medicine, Philadelphia, PA, USA

Eric R. Thuler, MD Robotic Surgery Center at Oswaldo Cruz German Hospital, São Paulo, Brazil

Department of ICEP, Hospital Sirio-Libanês, São Paulo, Brazil

Song Tar Toh, MBBS, MMED (ORL), FAMS (ORL) Department of Otolaryngology, Singapore General Hospital, Singapore, Singapore

Neil S. Tolley, MD, FRCS, DLO Department of Otorhinolaryngology and Head & Neck Surgery, St. Mary's Hospital, Imperial College Healthcare NHS Trust, London, UK

Fabiana C.P. Valera, MD, PhD Department of Ophthalmology, Otorhinolaryngology and Head and Neck Surgery, ENT Division, Medical School of Ribeirão Preto, University of São Paulo, Ribeirão Preto, Brazil

Tom Vauterin, MD Department of Otorhinolaryngology, Head and Neck Surgery, AZ Sint-Jan Bruges-Ostend, Brugge, Belgium

E. Vetri, MD Medical Direction, G.B. Morgagni—L. Pierantoni Hospital, Forlì, Italy

Claudio Vicini, MD Head and Neck Department - ENT & Oral Surgery Unit - G.B. Morgagni - L. Pierantoni Hospital, Forlì – Infermi Hospital, Faenza - ASL of Romagna, Italy

Jochen A. Werner, MD University Hospital of Essen, Essen, Germany

Claudia Zanotti, MD Head and Neck Department—ENT & Oral Surgery Unit, G.B. Morgagni–L. Pierantoni Hospital, ASL of Romagna, Forlì, Italy

Infermi Hospital, ASL of Romagna, Faenza, Italy

Ermelinda Zeccardo, MD Head and Neck Department—ENT & Oral Surgery Unit, G.B. Morgagni–L. Pierantoni Hospital, ASL of Romagna, Forlì, Italy

Infermi Hospital, ASL of Romagna, Faenza, Italy

Chapter 1
Introduction

Claudio Vicini, Filippo Montevecchi, and Paul T. Hoff

TORS for OSA (obstructive sleep apnea) is just one more of the many published applications of robotic surgery in the otolaryngology literature. The first case of TORS in humans for cancer was described by Weinstein et al. (2006). The first TORS for OSA was carried out in May 2008 in Forlì by Vicini and Montevecchi, with the cooperation of the first Forlì's ENT Robotic Team, including Dr. Giulia Tenti (staff member) and Pietro Canzi (senior resident). The surgery was planned after more than 1 year of training in Italy, France (IRCAD, Strasbourg), and the USA (Weinstein and O'Malley, Philadelphia, PA).

A 45-year-old truck driver suffering from moderate obstructive sleep apnea syndrome with a Apnea Hypopnea Index (AHI) of 27 related to enlarged lingual tonsils underwent a Trans-oral Robotic Tongue Base Reduction and Supraglottoplasty, deeply inspired by Chabolle's Tongue Base Reduction with Hyoid-Epiglottoplasty (TBRHE) procedure and by Weinstein–O'Malley's Trans-oral Robotic tongue base and supraglottic cancer resection. The overall surgical time was 60 min, no intraoperative or postoperative complications were registered, and the 6 months postoperative sleep study revealed an AHI of 2.

The first pilot series of TORS for OSA was reported by Vicini et al. 2 years later, in 2010. At that time the most effective codified tongue base (TB) procedure for moderate to severe OSA in Europe was Chabolle's operation, and in the USA the most popular approaches to TB reduction were either trans-oral endoscopic

C. Vicini, M.D. • F. Montevecchi, M.D. (✉)
Head and Neck Department - ENT & Oral Surgery Unit - G.B. Morgagni - L. Pierantoni Hospital, Forlì – Infermi Hospital, Faenza - ASL of Romagna, Italy
e-mail: claudio@claudiovicini.com; filippomontevecchi72@gmail.com

P.T. Hoff, M.S., M.D.
Department of Otolaryngology—Head and Neck Surgery, University of Michigan Hospital, Ann Arbor, MI, USA
e-mail: phoff@med.umich.edu

© Springer International Publishing Switzerland 2016

C. Vicini et al. (eds.), *TransOral Robotic Surgery for Obstructive Sleep Apnea*,
DOI 10.1007/978-3-319-34040-1_1

Coblation® resection or radiofrequency ablation. The literature of the previous 30 years is replete with more than 20 different solutions, with a wide latitude of technologies (cold and hot resection knives, lasers, radiofrequency tools, and a variety of suspension solutions including genioglossus advancement, suture suspensions, and more complex suspension devices). As usual when too many techniques are available, there is room for improvement. Obstructive sleep apnea syndrome is characterized by multilevel obstruction in a population with variable pharyngeal soft tissue anatomy, body mass index (BMI), and skeletal anatomy. No one technique will suit every patient.

The worldwide sleep surgery community continues to search for a new, perhaps more simple and effective solution. In 2009 a preliminary safety and feasibility study for TORS and OSA was carried out in a multi-center setting in Europe (Remacle—Belgium, Slama—Czech Republic, Kim—Korea, Krishnan—Australia, Vicini and Montevecchi—Italy). The picture (Fig. 1.1) includes all the members of the study team in Strasbourg, during the start-up meeting (2009). This study proved that TORS for OSA was a feasible procedure for managing tongue base obstruction with a negligible conversion rate from the planned surgery; more importantly the rate of significant complications was acceptably low. In the next couple of years an intense exchange of experience was registered, with USA surgeons (e.g. Thaler and Hoff) and Far East surgeons (Toh, Agrawal, etc.) as well as other European Centers. Many of the most expert North American Head & Neck Robotic Surgeons also shared their experience (Magnuson, Huntley, Holsinger and Duvvuri). In less than 10 years this application has spread all over the world, and the diffusion may be traced by the increasing number of published papers in the literature.

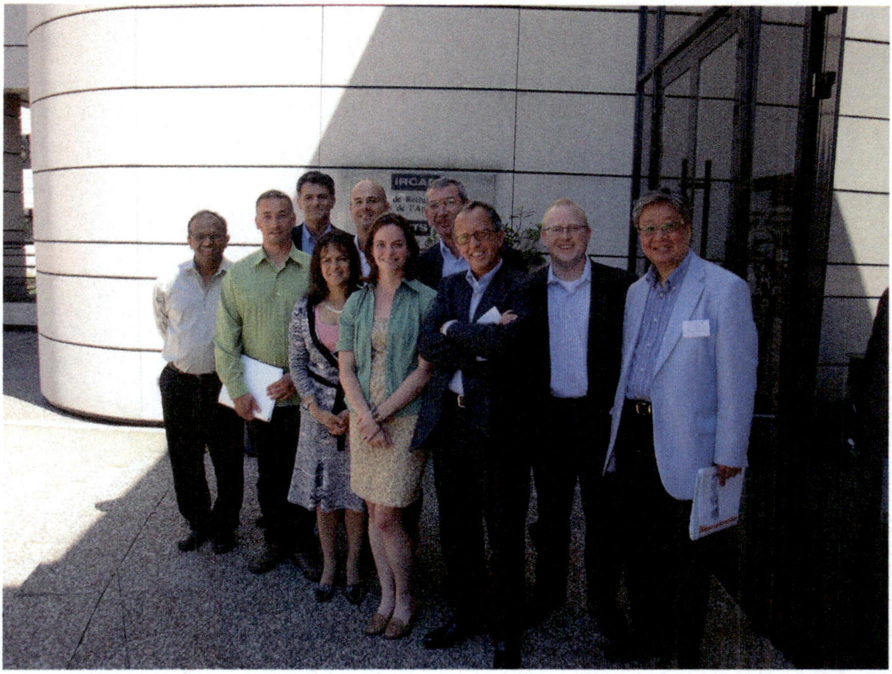

Fig. 1.1 The members of the TORS study in Strasbourg, France, during the start-up meeting (2009)

Part I
Patient Work-Up

Chapter 2
Tongue Pathophysiology in OSAS Patients: A Surgically Oriented Perspective

Filippo Montevecchi, Claudio Vicini, Matteo Costantini, Riccardo Gobbi, Elisabetta Firinu, Ottavio Piccin, and Giovanni Sorrenti

2.1 Introduction

The tongue is a complex organ composed of different groups of muscles, connective tissue, and fat deposits; it plays a central role in speech, deglutition, respiration, and the pathophysiology of obstructive sleep apnea (OSA) because of its direct involvement in the collapse of upper airway [1]. The tongue can be described in biomechanical terminology as a muscular hydrostat working within the framework of a rigid skeletal enclosure.

F. Montevecchi, M.D. (✉) • C. Vicini, M.D.
Head and Neck Department - ENT & Oral Surgery Unit - G.B. Morgagni - L. Pierantoni Hospital, Forlì – Infermi Hospital, Faenza - ASL of Romagna, Italy
e-mail: filo651@hotmail.com; filippomontevecchi72@gmail.com; claudio@claudiovicini.com

M. Costantini, M.D.
Department of Pathology, Head and Neck Department, Transfusion and Laboratory Medicine, G.B. Morgagni—L. Pierantoni Hospital, Via Carlo Forlanini, 34, Forlì 47121, Italy
e-mail: matteo.costantini@auslromagna.it

R. Gobbi, M.D. • E. Firinu, M.D.
Head and Neck Department—ENT & Oral Surgery Unit, G.B. Morgagni—L. Pierantoni Hospital, Forli - Infermi Hospital, Faenza - ASL of Romagna, Italy
e-mail: DR.RICCARDOGOBBI@GMAIL.COM; elisabetta.firinu@libero.it

O. Piccin, M.D., M.Sc • G. Sorrenti, M.D.
Otolaryngoloy and Audiology Unit, Head and Neck Surgery, Sant'Orsola-Malpighi Hospital, Bologna University, Via G.Massarenti 9, Bologna 40138, Italy
e-mail: ottavio.piccin@gmail.com; gisorrenti@yahoo.it

© Springer International Publishing Switzerland 2016

C. Vicini et al. (eds.), *TransOral Robotic Surgery for Obstructive Sleep Apnea*,
DOI 10.1007/978-3-319-34040-1_2

2.2 Anatomy of the Human Tongue (Table 2.1)

The human tongue can be anatomically divided into three parts:

1. the Blade or tip, which is the region anterior to the frenulum
2. the Body, which extends from the frenulum anteriorly to the circumvallate papillae posteriorly
3. the Base (BOT), posterior to the circumvallate papillae.

The musculature of the tongue is composed by several interweaving groups of muscles that are divided in two groups by their origins and insertions. This architecture gives the tongue its characteristics of strength and dexterity.

The extrinsic muscles have a bony insertion, while the other end inserts within the tongue musculature; in contrast, the intrinsic muscles have no bony insertions and all muscular insertions are within the tongue. The extrinsic muscles primarily move the tongue, whereas the intrinsic muscles alter the shape of the tongue.

In the following paragraphs the intrinsic and extrinsic muscles are described in detail.

The intrinsic muscles are the Superior Longitudinal (SL), Inferior Longitudinal (IL), Transverse (T), and Vertical (V) muscles.

The SL is a longitudinally oriented muscular sheet with a high representation of connective tissue that occupies the length of the tongue. The SL muscle is located immediately deep to the superior mucosal surface of the tongue. The muscle is thin in the anterior tongue and becomes progressively thicker toward the BOT; its function is to both shorten the tongue and dorsiflex the tip.

The IL muscle originates close to BOT and hyoid bone and is composed of a larger oblique component that spans from the BOT to the blade of the tongue; a

Table 2.1 Muscles of the human tongue

Muscles	Actions	Insertions
Genioglossus	Tongue protrusion, hyoid bone anteriorization, tongue body depression, tongue tip dorsiflexion and retrusion	Genial tuberosity of the mandible, tongue length, hyoid bone
Hyoglossus	Tongue depression and retraction	Hyoid bone, tongue length
Styloglossus	Tongue retrusion and elevation	Styloid process, stylomandibular ligament
Palatoglossus	–	Soft palate's aponeurosis
Glossopharyngeus	–	Inferior part of superior pharyngeal constrictor
Superior Longitudinal	Tongue shortening and dorsiflexion	Submucous fibrous layer
Inferior Longitudinal	Tongue shortening and retroflexion	Tongue base
Transverse	Tongue narrowing and elongating	Median septum
Vertical	Tongue flattening and broadening	Genioglossus

smaller horizontal part of the IL is situated in the tongue blade. Contraction of IL results in tongue shortening and retro-flexion.

The Transverse muscle (T) originates from the median septum and courses laterally toward the lateral connective tissue of the tongue surface. Its actions are to narrow and elongate the tongue body and blade. The Vertical (V) is the final major intrinsic muscle, an extension of the genioglossal muscle (GG) in the medial third of the body of the tongue, and its function is to flatten and broaden the tongue.

The extrinsic muscles are described below:

The GG is often considered both an intrinsic and extrinsic muscle. From the genial tuberosity to the hyoid bone the GG is composed of three distinct sections defined by the orientation of the muscle fascicles. The Anterior fascicles are vertically oriented, and are responsible for dorsiflexion and retrusion of the tongue tip. Posteriorly the GG fascicles become wider and oblique as they approach the BOT where the fascicles assume a horizontal orientation before inserting in to the hyoid bone. The main role of the GG is protrusion of the tongue through the action of the posterior fascicles together with the anterior movement of the hyoid bone during the inspiration.

The Hyoglossus muscle (HG) originates from the body of the greater cornu of the hyoid bone after which it fans out horizontally and inserts along the length of the tongue. The action of HG is to retrude and depress the lateral margin of the tongue.

The Styloglossus (SG) is a small, thin muscle that originates from the styloid process and the stylomandibular ligament. It is the most lateral of the tongue muscles and its function is to retrude and elevate the lateral margin of the tongue [1, 2].

The hypoglossal nerve provides innervation to both the intrinsic and extrinsic muscles of the tongue. The contraction of this nerve enables a variety of movements including protrusion, and stiffening of the tongue as well as enlarging of the upper airway during wakefulness and sleep.

Neuropathic damage to the tongue musculature (especially the GG) may occur due to REM-associated hypotonia, snoring-related trauma, aging, and hypoxia due to repeated apneic episodes; this may lead to an increased tendency toward upper airway collapse.

2.3 Characteristics of the Tongue in Awake Patient

The tongue is one of the main contributors in the pathophysiology of multilevel upper airways (UAW) collapse in OSAS patients. The anatomical and functional complexity of the tongue including deglutition, airway maintenance, and speech has been described in different geometrical models [2].

The lingual tonsils are part of the ring of lymphoid tissue (Waldeyer's ring) that lines the nasopharynx and oropharynx. Lingual tonsil hypertrophy can contribute to upper airway obstruction and has been associated with laryngopharyngeal reflux, reactive lymphoid hyperplasia due to previous adeno-tonsillectomy, obesity, smoking and pharmacology (phenytoin) [3]. In particular it has been demonstrated that in OSAS patients lingual tonsil hypertrophy grade is significantly related with laryngopharyngeal reflux, smoking and younger age; on the contrary there are still opposing data about correlation between BMI and lingual tonsil hypertrophy [3–5].

In anatomic study of lingual fat conducted in general population at autopsy a higher percentage of fat deposition was found in tongue muscle compared to other somatic muscles; furthermore, the study showed a topographic distribution of fat deposits with the largest accumulation of fat found in the posterior third of the tongue (BOT) and in the sublingual region (below the intrinsic tongue muscles and interdigitated within the genioglossus fibers). The percentage of fat in the tongue, especially in the posterior portion, was found to be positively correlated with BMI and with tongue weight [6]. Further study in overweigh and obese patients confirmed the preferential deposition of fat in the base of tongue, and demonstrated a higher percentage of fat in apneic compared to non-apneic patients. It is now clear that tongue volume, and lingual fat percentage are greater in obese apneic patients than in obese non-apneic patients.

Furthermore, the additional presence of intramuscular fat tissue infiltration, rather than isolated fat deposits, may interfere with muscle contraction leading to a decrease in the performance of the tongue as pharyngeal dilator muscle [7].

2.4 Characteristics of the Tongue During Sleep

Because upper airway obstruction and apnea are dynamic processes, analysis of the anatomical changes that occur during natural sleep or drug induced sedation is mandatory.

In the OSAS patient there are different characteristic alterations in the position and size of the tongue; sedated MRI studies have shown retrodisplacement of the anterior and posterior tongue in OSAS patients as compared to normal controls [8, 9]. Others have demonstrated a reduction in the retrolingual space in patients with nasal obstruction; this shift to oral breathing causes a backward movement of the soft palate against the posterior pharyngeal wall and posterior inferior positioning of the mandible and tongue with narrowing of the posterior airway space [10]. REM sleep is associated with marked hypotonia and subsequent worsening of OSAS due to collapse of the tongue and associated pharyngeal dilators [9].

2.5 Final Remarks

Many surgical treatments for tongue base obstruction in patients with OSA have been described in literature. Careful assessment of the specific pattern of tongue base narrowing may have a crucial impact on the selection of the correct therapy for every patient. Current surgical procedures are designed to affect the volumetric expansion of the airway based on the findings identified both in the office and during sedated endoscopy; these include lymphoid hypertrophy, muscular hypertrophy, nasal obstruction and oral breathing, retroposition of the tongue. Patients may be presented a variety of treatment choices including multilevel surgery, hypoglossal nerve stimulation, oral appliance therapy or medical weight loss.

Taking into account the anatomical and pathophysiological characteristics of the tongue, both in sleep and awake conditions, should provide a reasonable guide to an appropriate surgical choice for the treatment of the tongue.

A complete evaluation of the patient, including imaging studies during wakefulness, such as cephalometry and/or CT/MRI, and sleep, properly DISE, can be helpful in better understanding the complexities of the upper airway [11].

References

1. Sanders I, Mu L. A three-dimensional atlas of human tongue muscles. Anat Rec (Hoboken). 2013;296(7):1102–14.
2. Kjajee Y, Pelteret J-PV, et al. The biomechanics of the human tongue. Int J Numer Method Biomed Eng. 2013;29:492–514.
3. Kim AM, Keenan BT, Jackson N, Chan EL, Staley B, Poptani H, et al. Tongue fat and its relationship to obstructive sleep apnea. Sleep. 2014;37(10):1639–48.
4. Nashi N, Kang S, Barkdull GC, Lucas J, Davidson TM. Lingual fat at autopsy. Laryngoscope. 2007;117:1467–73.
5. Sung MW, Lee WH, Wee JH, et al. Factors associated with hypertrophy of the lingual tonsils in adults with sleep-disordered breathing. JAMA Otolaryngol Head Neck Surg. 2013;139:598–603.
6. Hwang MS, Salapatas AM, Yalamanchali S, Joseph NJ, Friedman M. Factors associated with hypertrophy of the lingual tonsils. Otolaryngol Head Neck Surg. 2015;152(5):851–5.
7. Moore KE, Phillips C. A practical method for describing patterns of tongue-base narrowing (modification of Fujita) in awake adult patients with obstructive sleep apnea. J Oral Maxillofac Surg. 2002;60(3):252–60.
8. Wang Y, Mcdonald JP, Liu Y, Pan K, Zhang X, Hu R. Dynamic alterations of the tongue in obstructive sleep apnea-hypopnea syndrome during sleep: analysis using ultrafast MRI. Genet Mol Res. 2014;13(2):4552–63.
9. McSharry DG, Saboisky JP, DeYoung P, Jordan AS, Trinder J, Smales E, et al. Physiological mechanisms of upper airway hypotonia during REM sleep. Sleep. 2014;37(3):561–9.
10. Lee SHL, Choi JH, Shin C, Lee HM, Kwon SY, Lee SH. How does open-mouth breathing influence upper airway anatomy. Laryngoscope. 2007;117:1102–6.
11. Eckert DJ, Malhotra A. Pathophysiology of adult obstructive sleep apnea. Proc Am Thorac Soc. 2008;5(2):144–53.

Chapter 3
History-Taking and Clinical Examination

Claudio Vicini, Filippo Montevecchi, Paul T. Hoff, Claudia Zanotti, Tod Huntley, and Yassin Bahgat

3.1 Introduction

A complete history, head and neck physical examination, and upper airway flexible endoscopy are mandatory in the clinical approach to any patient with OSA being considered for robotic surgery. The initial office encounter will provide crucial information including patient expectations, polysomnography results, subjective measures of daytime fatigue and swallowing function, as well as anatomic characteristics such as lymphoid tissue hypertrophy, muscular tongue hypertrophy, elongated or narrow palate, and nasal obstruction. This data is integrated and provides both the

C. Vicini, M.D. • F. Montevecchi, M.D. (✉)
Head and Neck Department - ENT & Oral Surgery Unit - G.B. Morgagni - L. Pierantoni Hospital, Forlì – Infermi Hospital, Faenza - ASL of Romagna, Forlì, Italy
e-mail: claudio@claudiovicini.com; filo651@hotmail.com; filippomontevecchi72@gmail.com

P. Hoff, M.S., M.D.
Department of Otolaryngology—Head and Neck Surgery, University of Michigan, 1500 East Medical Center Drive, Ann Arbor, MI 48109, USA

C. Zanotti, M.D.
Head and Neck Department—ENT & Oral Surgery Unit, G.B. Morgagni–L. Pierantoni Hospital, ASL of Romagna, Forlì, Italy

Infermi Hospital, ASL of Romagna, Faenza, Italy
e-mail: zanotti.claudia89@gmail.com

T. Huntley, M.D., F.A.C.S.
CENTA: Center for Ear Nose Throat & Allergy, 12188—A North Meridian Street, Suite 375, Carmel, IN 46032, USA
e-mail: thuntley@centadocs.com

Y. Bahgat, M.D., M.Sc., E.B.E.
Department of Otorhinolaryngology—Head & Neck Surgery, Alexandria University, Alexandria, Egypt
e-mail: yassinbahgat@hotmail.com

© Springer International Publishing Switzerland 2016

C. Vicini et al. (eds.), *TransOral Robotic Surgery for Obstructive Sleep Apnea*, DOI 10.1007/978-3-319-34040-1_3

patient and surgeon confidence in deciding to offer TORS multilevel surgery or, alternatively, to suggest alternative treatments both operative and nonoperative.

If properly applied, the history and physical examination may provide the surgeon with important information about candidacy for surgery including:

1. Are the patient's complaints consistent with OSA or is there another unrelated cause of Sleep Disordered Breathing (SDB) that may be addressed without surgery?
2. Are there findings during the history and physical examination that may provide preliminary information about the presence and severity of OSA in patients who have not undergone previous PSG?
3. Can the site(s) of obstruction be determined by history and physical examination in the awake, non-sedated office setting?
4. Is it possible to identify candidates for TORS based on a pathological profile beginning with the office examination and then confirmed with DISE?
5. On the contrary, are there clinical findings that exclude patients from consideration for TORS?
6. Are there anatomic predictors that determine adequate exposure to successfully perform TORS?
7. Are there predictors of success (Predictive index) that will guide surgeons to select appropriate candidates for TORS?

3.2 The New Concept of OSA Patient Phenotype

The concept of phenotyping OSA patients is a new and effective way of integrating both the history and physical exam to determine eligibility for TORS. In a simple clinical setting a long list of "*anatomical phenotypes*" may be described as well a wide variety of "*psychological phenotypes*", both of paramount importance for a correct patient selection. A more complete set of data, described as "*functional phenotypes*" are available during the next step of evaluation, during drug induced sedated endoscopy (DISE), and will be discussed in detail in Chap. 7. In Fig. 3.1 a list of the most useful clinical phenotype is summarized. In addition to basic information about the patients pathology, phenotyping provides the surgeon with a reliable tool for collecting sound data about exposure challenges and about the expected outcomes.

During routine office evaluation, including flexible fiber-optic endoscopy, the observed anatomy may disclose one of two phenotypes: multilevel or single level obstruction. Many classification systems are available for describing and scoring the affected sites during both office examination and DISE including the degree of obstruction and the pattern of collapse. There is no single correct staging system that has been endorsed and different systems may be used to visualize and describe possible sites of obstruction in an ordered fashion (VOTE [1], NOHL [2]). Multilevel obstructive phenotypes include cases in which nasal obstruction is associated with oropharyngeal obstruction (palate and palatine tonsils) and lateral wall, tongue

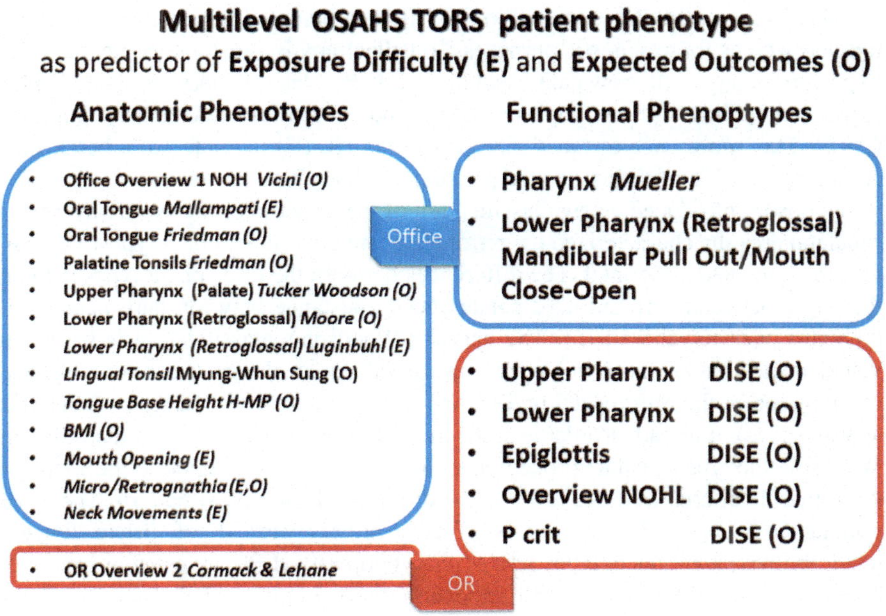

Fig. 3.1 The list of the most useful clinical phenotypes

base, and/or supraglottic collapse. Multilevel collapse requires planning for a multilevel procedure instead of a single level procedure, which implies a more invasive procedure, a longer operative time, as well as a more difficult postoperative period for the patient. Outcomes following multilevel surgery, including TORS, are superior to single level surgery in properly selected patients [3].

Michael Friedman modified the Mallampati score [4] by characterizing tongue/palate in a tongue-in instead of tongue-out position on direct inspection [5]. Tongue-in Friedman score III to IV describe a huge body of the tongue. It strongly relates to a possible important role of the oral tongue instead of the pharyngeal tongue (tongue base) in the overall tongue obstruction. This finding was classically used as a warning for the surgeon about the possible failure if a single level palate procedure such as uvulopalatopharyngoplasty (UP3) is planned without addressing the tongue, especially in overweight/obese patients. Friedman's tongue palate classification system may also be important in planning anterior midline glossectomy as an additional procedure after tongue base reduction, if required. Conceptually, lingual hypertrophy (macroglossia) may not only be located at the base of the tongue, but may cause obstruction due to oral tongue hypertrophy. The tongue must be considered in its entirety; Friedman score may help to defined this fundamental feature. Patients with a Friedman tongue/palate score of 3–4 may fail in case of pure tongue base reduction and the surgeon must consider the possibility of a more extended lingualplasty including an anterior midline glossectomy. In cases of anterior midline glossectomy a two stage operation may be necessary and airway management may include tracheostomy.

Tonsil size scoring (Friedman 0 to IV) [6] must be noted for planning tonsillectomy as well as for prognostic purposes. Tonsillectomy is a mandatory step in order to perform many of the new palate techniques such as lateral pharyngoplasty (LPh), expansion sphincter pharyngoplasty (ESP), and barbed relocation pharyngoplasty (BRP). The importance of tonsil size (Friedman III, IV) is related to a better outcome, irrespective of the associated palate procedure [7].

Woodson introduced a new classification of the upper pharyngeal airway or retropalatal area; he characterized the retropalatal area into three phenotypes: vertical, intermediate, and horizontal. The differences between the three phenotypes include the angle between soft and hard palate and the distance between hard palate and posterior pharyngeal wall [8]. The data for Woodson's classification is based on visual inspection of the oropharynx, transnasal upper airway flexible endoscope examination of the retropalatal region, and from the lateral cephalogram (posterior airway space), if already available at the time of the first consultation. According to Woodson, the type of palate procedure technique should be adapted to the shape of the retropalatal area in order to fit to the different phenotypical pattern. The most popular UP3 is probably much less effective in very vertical soft palate. For the most oblique palate phenotypes lateral pharyngoplasty (LPh), expansion sphincter pharyngoplasty (ESP) and barbed relocation pharyngoplasty (BRP) may be more appropriate. Transpalatal advancement pharyngoplasty [9] is probably the best choice in vertical phenotype with long hard palates. This relative new and smart way of phenotyping the retropalatal area is of paramount importance for planning the best associated palate procedure.

The lower pharyngeal airway is more commonly described as the retrolingual space. The lower pharyngeal space may be reduced by an inward collapse of the lateral wall or by a posterior collapse of the tongue base. Moore introduced a morphological classification according to the vertical location of tongue base obstruction: prevalent obstruction at the superior aspect of the tongue base (Type A), diffuse obstruction (Type B), prevalent obstruction at the lower aspect of the tongue base (Type C) [10]. These different retrolingual phenotypes are easily recognized by a simple flexible fiber-optic inspection of the retrolingual space with the patient in upright position, during Mueller maneuver, and with the patient lying down. This classification system is of practical importance for planning the best surgical procedure, and for obtaining a simple preoperative outcomes index. The most favorable type of obstruction for TORS is Moore Type C with a prevalence of obstruction at the lower aspect of tongue base. On the other hand the less suitable patient for TORS is described by a phenotype including a very high, vertical and muscular tongue base, with a very thin lingual tonsil (Moore type A and B).

The Moore phenotypes can be easily identified during fiber-optic examination where the distance between the circumvallate papilla and the vallecula is elongated (high vertical face). If a lateral cephalogram is available, the tongue base height may be easily visualized; a high vertical tongue usually correlates to a mandible plane to hyoid (MPH) greater than 35 mm. Patients with an MPH greater than 35 mm are not good candidates for TORS tongue base reduction. On the contrary, patients with an

MPH less than 35 mm and Moore type C tongue base anatomy may benefit from multilevel surgery including TORS for retrolingual obstruction.

Patients with a posterior airway space (PAS) less than 10 mm have inferior outcomes following stand-alone UP3 [11]. These patients often require additional tongue base procedure to achieve a successful outcome.

The importance of lingual tonsil hypertrophy has long been recognized as a significant factor in OSA, but only recently with the advent of TORS do sleep surgeons have a tool that can effectively and safely manage this pathology in retrolingual region. Friedman and Myung Sung have recently provided details of lingual tonsil hypertrophy including practical classification systems [12, 13]. In our experience massive and diffuse lingual tonsil hypertrophy requiring a wide lingual tonsillectomy is associated with more favorable outcomes. Lingual tonsil hypertrophy phenotypes allow the surgeon to remove a significant amount of obstructing tissue with minimal morbidity and without violation of the underlying muscle. Lingual tonsil volume is a reliable prognostic index. The best candidates for TORS, especially for the novice surgeon, are those patients with localized, low, lymphoid tongue base obstruction (the triple-L).

Body mass index (kg/m^2) is easily calculated and provides important information about candidacy for surgery. In our protocol for multilevel surgery of the upper airway patients with a BMI over 35 are excluded from consideration. Below this value, BMI may be used as prognostic index for success. According to Forlì Hospital data (unpublished data), in a retrospective study comparing matched pairs of patients treated by TORS or maxillomandibular advancement, robotic surgery proved to be as effective as facial bone framework surgery if BMI < 30 and less effective if BMI > 30. Hoff et al. published a paper dealing with BMI and TORS outcomes, where the findings are similar [14].

Patient selection is dependent not only on phenotypic characteristics that are predictors of success, but also is dependent on reliable of information about the expected probability of obtaining sufficient surgical field exposure. Adequate exposure allows for better outcomes related to:

1. The ability to remove obstructing tissue which is related to successful reduction of AHI
2. Prevention of complications such as pharyngeal stenosis
3. The ability to manage complications such as bleeding should they occur. Poor visualization of important anatomic structures may result in inadvertent injury to neurovascular structures and late circular scaring of the lateral and posterior hypopharyngeal walls.

The first basic prerequisite for any transoral surgical procedure is the degree of mouth opening, usually expressed as inter-incisive distance (cm) during maximal active opening of the mouth. In most of TORS patients the inter-incisive distance is more than 4 cm. The lower limit of opening required for a safe intubation, as described by Gupta [15] is at least 2 cm. Inter-incisive distance is much more important for the bedside assistant than for the console surgeon. It is not difficult to place the 8 mm scope and 5 mm instruments in to a narrow oral aperture with an inter-incisor distance as low as 2 cm, however this reduced access may impede the ability of the assistant to retract and control bleeding, making the surgery more difficult and dangerous.

The well-known Mallampati score (tongue out instead of tongue in as described by Friedman classification) as used by anesthesiologists in determining intubation difficulty may be a very useful phenotype to the TORS surgeon as well. A Mallampati type III or IV describes a huge oral tongue phenotype. In the TORS setting a high tongue body dorsum may produce significant difficulties in the tongue base exposure, which often result in less tissue removal (worse outcomes) and higher probability of posterior wall injury (higher probability of late postoperative strictures).

The use of imaging may also aid the surgeon in determining the likelihood of suitable exposure for TORS. Evaluation of the lateral cephalogram or CT/MRI, as described in the imaging chapter, will clearly define the posterior airway space (PAS) as well as the presence or absence of retrognathia and the vertical height of the tongue base by assessing the distance of the mandibular plane to the hyoid (MPH). These simple measurements may offer a very reliable favorability index for TORS exposure [16].

Micro and/or retrognathia phenotypes are usually evident without imaging and can be determined during a general examination using the Angle's classification system; however, additional more quantitative information may come from lateral cephalogram evaluation. Severe degrees of retrognathia are better managed using skeletal framework surgery (maxillomandibular advancement, which must be offered to the patient as an alternative to TORS). Less severe retrognathia cases may be approached with a reasonable expectation for success, however, the surgeon must be prepared for a more difficult exposure and less predictable results even in patients with localized, low, lymphoid tissue "triple L." A normal tongue body volume in patients with retrognathia may be more difficult to fit into a narrow mandibular angle during exposure, which may require increased blade pressure, potentially threatening the lingual nerve function resulting in hypesthesia and dysgeusia.

At the time of the first clinical consultation the experienced sleep surgeon should pay close attention to the intentions, expectations, and personality of the patients considering alternatives to conservative therapy. This collected data may be defined as the "*psychological phenotype*." The psychologic phenotype includes a wide range of different and loosely defined features, including:

1. *Patient's OSA awareness profile*. The patient perception of OSA may range from a complete unawareness of the problem (no daytime symptoms) to the group of sleepy patients with cognitive or sexual impairment, or with previous cardiovascular episodes related to OSA. Some patients suffer from repeated episodes of nighttime choking episodes that awakening them from sleep.
2. *Patients motivation profile*. Motivation is dependent upon both subjective symptoms and objective signs or sequela of OSA. Some patients may accept improvement where others will only accept cure of OSA. It is important that the patient understand that there is a difference between improvement in symptoms and the ability to discontinue CPAP. Not all patients who undergo TORS multilevel surgery are able to discontinue CPAP.

3. *Patient's previous treatment history*. All patients who undergo TORS should have had a trial of CPAP. Patients who have failed CPAP may have different expectation than those who have failed previous surgical attempts.
4. *The "happy snorer" psychological phenotype* depicts a middle age male, not aware of the OSA severity, referred (forced to the consultation) by the bed partner, concerned only for the relational impact of the snoring. The level of motivation is usually low, surgery acceptance low, and the risk of postoperative functional complaints is usually very high.
5. *The "sleepy patient"* is by far the preferred candidate for TORS, because he/she is usually aware of the impact of OSA on daily life, and the usual perceived positive effect of surgery on daytime sleepiness may compensate for minimal possible side effects.
6. *The "asymptomatic severe OSA patient"* presents a significant challenge for the surgeon. These patients are typically referred by the pulmonologist/neurologist after CPAP failure. The patient's lack of a perceived health problem may reduce the level of motivation and the acceptance rate of a surgical alternative.
7. *The "choking patient"* may be defined as patients who, irrespective of the degree of OSA severity, complain of repeated bouts of nocturnal sudden awakening with a sensation of suffocation and impending death. The condition is not really life threatening, but it makes the patient acutely aware of OSA in a dramatic way, stressing the need for a quick and effective remedy, including surgery.
8. *The "psychiatric patient"* encompasses a wide range of possible associated psychopathological conditions not related to OSA. The most common situations include anxiety, panic attacks, and depression states. In the well-known Stanford Protocol any recognized psychiatric condition must be considered as a relative contra-indication to surgery. In anxious and depressed subjects the immediate post-op period may be difficult to manage and may result in an exacerbation of the underlying symptomatology. Patients with psychiatric disorders are at increased risk to complain about side effects (globus, altered taste, pain) usually well tolerated or accepted by other patients.
9. *The "Munchausen patient"* is not common, but on the other hand not immediately easy to identify. This patient describes a significant history of many previous failed surgeries for OSA. It is interesting that in many cases the previous surgeries are reported in great detail, but the relative pre-op and post-op sleep studies are missing or overlooked. For this kind of patients any innovative and futuristic surgical technology, namely robotic surgery, is very attractive or irresistible. It is our strong feeling that this kind of patient must be discouraged from surgery and referred to a psychiatrist for proper treatment.
10. *The "patient already surgically treated but failed"* is a special psychological phenotype. Usually the patient is referred from a sleep medicine colleague after a postoperative polysomnogram demonstrates persistent OSA, or a patient self refers with persistent symptoms of excessive daytime somnolence. These patients may feel that robotic surgery is their last chance for a cure. That patient is exploring surgery as an option reflects their commitment to finding relief of persistent symptoms; this problem is a high priority. In our experience the best

approach to these patients is to present all options (surgical and nonsurgical) and to assure the patient that a thorough evaluation will be performed in order to understand whether or not he or she is a candidate for surgery.

References

1. Kezirian EJ, Hohenhorst W, de Vries N. Drug-induced sleep endoscopy: the VOTE classification. Eur Arch Otorhinolaryngol. 2011;268(8):1233–6.
2. Vicini C, De Vito A, Benazzo M, Frassineti S, Campanini A, Frasconi P, Mira E. The nose oropharynx hypopharynx and larynx (NOHL) classification: a new system of diagnostic standardized examination for OSAHS patients. Eur Arch Otorhinolaryngol. 2012;269(4): 1297–300.
3. Thaler ER, Rassekh CH, Lee JM, Weinstein GS, O'Malley Jr BW. Outcomes for multilevel surgery for sleep apnea: obstructive sleep apnea, transoral robotic surgery, and uvulopalatopharyngoplasty. Laryngoscope. 2015 Jul 7. doi:10.1002/lary.25353 [Epub ahead of print].
4. Mallampati SR, Gatt SP, Gugino LD, Desai SP, Waraksa B, Freiberger D, Liu PL. A clinical sign to predict difficult tracheal intubation: a prospective study. Can Anaesth Soc J. 1985;32(4):429–34.
5. Friedman M, Hamilton C, Samuelson CG, Lundgren ME, Pott T. Diagnostic value of the Friedman tongue position and Mallampati classification for obstructive sleep apnea: a meta-analysis. Otolaryngol Head Neck Surg. 2013;148(4):540–7.
6. Friedman M, Tanyeri H, La Rosa M, Landsberg R, Vaidyanathan K, Pieri S, Caldarelli D. Clinical predictors of obstructive sleep apnea. Laryngoscope. 1999;109(12):1901–7.
7. Senchak AJ, McKinlay AJ, Acevedo J, Swain B, Tiu MC, Chen BS, Robitschek J, Ruhl DS, Williams LL, Camacho M, Frey WC, O'Connor PD. The effect of tonsillectomy alone in adult obstructive sleep apnea. Otolaryngol Head Neck Surg. 2015;152(5):969–73.
8. Woodson BT. A method to describe the pharyngeal airway. Laryngoscope. 2015;125(5): 1233–8.
9. Woodson BT, Robinson S, Lim HJ. Transpalatal advancement pharyngoplasty outcomes compared with uvulopalatopharygoplasty. Otolaryngol Head Neck Surg. 2005;133(2):211–7.
10. Moore KE, Phillips C. A practical method for describing patterns of tongue-base narrowing (modification of Fujita) in awake adult patients with obstructive sleep apnea. J Oral Maxillofac Surg. 2002;60(3):252–60. discussion 260–1.
11. Lyberg T, Krogstad O, Djupesland G. Cephalometric analysis in patients with obstructive sleep apnoea syndrome: II. Soft tissue morphology. J Laryngol Otol. 1989;103(3):293–7.
12. Friedman M, Yalamanchali S, Gorelick G, Joseph NJ, Hwang MS. A standardized lingual tonsil grading system: interexaminer agreement. Otolaryngol Head Neck Surg. 2015;152(4):667–72.
13. Sung MW, Lee WH, Wee JH, Lee CH, Kim E, Kim JW. Factors associated with hypertrophy of the lingual tonsils in adults with sleep-disordered breathing. JAMA Otolaryngol Head Neck Surg. 2013;139(6):598–603.
14. Hoff PT, Glazer TA, Spector ME. Body mass index predicts success in patients undergoing transoral robotic surgery for obstructive sleep apnea. ORL J Otorhinolaryngol Relat Spec. 2014;76(5):266–72.
15. Gupta S, Sharma KR, Jain D. Airway assessment predictors of difficult airway. Indian J Anaesth. 2005;49(4):257–62.
16. Luginbuhl A, Baker A, Curry J, Drejet S, Miller M, Cognetti D. Preoperative cephalometric analysis to predict transoral robotic surgery exposure. J Robot Surg. 2014;8(4):313–7 [Epub 2014 Jun 24].

Chapter 4
Sleep Studies

Brian W. Rotenberg, Marcello Bosi, Sabrina Frassineti, and Venerino Poletti

4.1 Introduction

Sleep-related breathing disorders (SBD) are included in the International Classification of Sleep Disorders [1], and, more specifically, obstructive sleep apnea syndrome (OSAS) is the most common. OSAS is defined as a combination of some comorbidities and/or symptoms (such as excessive sleepiness, cognitive-behavioral) plus repeated episodes of upper airway obstruction during sleep.

A diagnosis of OSAS incorporates elements of history and physical findings, but also typically includes polysomongraphy (PSG) that measures most importantly the apnea/hypopnea index (AHI) reflecting the number of apneas and hypopneas per hour of sleep.

B.W. Rotenberg, M.D., M.P.H., F.R.C.S.C. (✉)
Department of Otolaryngology—Head & Neck Surgery, Western University,
268 Grosvenor Street, London, ON, Canada, N6A 4V2
e-mail: drbwrotenberg@sjhc.london.on.ca

M. Bosi, M.D.
Pulmonary Operative Unit, Department of Thoracic Diseases, G.B. Morgagni–L. Pierantoni Hospital, Via Carlo Forlanini, 34, 47121 Forlì, Italy

S. Frassineti, M.D.
Head and Neck Department—ENT & Oral Surgery Unit, G.B. Morgagni–L. Pierantoni Hospital, ASL of Romagna, Forlì, Italy

Infermi Hospital, ASL of Romagna, Faenza, Italy
e-mail: s.frassineti@libero.it

V. Poletti, M.D.
Pulmonary Operative Unit, Department of Thoracic Diseases, G.B. Morgagni–L. Pierantoni Hospital, Via Carlo Forlanini, 34, 47121 Forlì, Italy

Department of Respiratory Diseases & Allergology, Aarhus University Hospital, Aarhus, Denmark
e-mail: venerino.poletti@gmail.com

© Springer International Publishing Switzerland 2016
C. Vicini et al. (eds.), *TransOral Robotic Surgery for Obstructive Sleep Apnea*,
DOI 10.1007/978-3-319-34040-1_4

OSAS is diagnosed by [1]:

- an AHI >5 obstructive events per hour measured by PSG associated with comorbidities or symptoms that are related to the disease and unexplained by any other causes.
- an AHI >15 obstructive events per hour.

This definition can be controversial because considering an AHI of >5 or >15 events/h as abnormal is arguable and it is probable that the threshold for abnormality differs in accordance with sex and age.

4.2 Classification of Sleep Studies

An attended PSG evaluation involving monitoring of both sleep and respiration is considered standard practice for diagnosis of suspected OSAS, but a comprehensive sleep history and physical examination remains the cornerstone of the initial evaluation of any patient with sleep-related complaints. A number of sleep disorders can be diagnosed solely on the basis of a clinical evaluation and do not require a PSG.

In 1994, the American Association of Sleep Medicine (AASM) [2] classified sleep studies into four types, based on the number and types of physiological variables recorded and the presence or absence of attending personnel (Table 4.1).

Levels 2–3–4 were introduced as a more accessible and less expensive alternative to in-laboratory polysomnography. Unlike level 1–2, levels 3 and 4 testing

Table 4.1 Types of sleep studies (6-h overnight recording minimum)

	Type 1	Type 2	Type 3	Type 4
Number of leads	≥7 (generally > 16)	≥7	≥4	1–2
Types of leads	EEG, EOG, EMG, ECG, airflow, effort, oximetry	EEG, EOG, EMG, ECG, airflow, effort, oximetry	ECG, airflow, effort, oximetry (at least two channels are respiratory movements or respiratory movement and airflow)	Oximetry and other (usually airflow)
Body position	Objectively measured	Optional	Optional	Not measured
Setting	Attended	Unattended	Attended or unattended	Attended or unattended
Description	Standard PSG performed in a sleep laboratory	Comprehensive portable PSG	Portable testing limited to sleep apnea	Continuous recording of oxygen sat

cannot measure the duration of sleep, the number of arousals or sleep stages, nor can it detect nonrespiratory sleep disorders. More recently the SCOPER categorization system (Table 4.2), a new categorization system for portable monitoring devices [3] has been proposed based on measurements of sleep (S), cardiovascular (C), oximetry (O), position (P), effort (E), and respiratory parameters (R).

4.3 PSG-Level 1 and AASM Practice Parameters

Attended PSG records the physiological signals to quantify sleep, sleep disorders and associated events during sleep in order to achieve a diagnosis as defined in the third edition of the International Classification of Sleep Disorders [1]. Sleep scoring recordings have to include the electroencephalogram (EEG), left and right electro-oculogram (EOG), and the chin electromyogram (EMG). The recording of respiratory function requires assessment of oronasal airflow, the assessment of the thorax and abdomen movements, and the assessment of ventilation and blood gas. For nocturnal respiratory events definitions for apnea and hypopnea of the different types are given, and there are two definitions for hypopnea (recommended and acceptable). To distinguish obstructive and central respiratory events, respiratory inductive plethysmography is recognized as providing acceptable results [4]. In order to recognize periods of hypoventilation during sleep, carbon dioxide is quantitatively recorded [4]. Snoring sounds are recorded with the help of a pharyngeal microphone. Motor activities, such as periodic leg movements, bruxism and rapid eye movements (REM) sleep-behavior disorders are also clearly defined [4].

4.3.1 Scoring Respiratory Events

The American Academy of Sleep Medicine (AASM) has standardized PSG scoring over time, with the latest guidelines [4] defining an apnea as a cessation of airflow for a minimum of 10 s based on a thermal sensor and a reference sensor (Fig. 4.1) and an hypopnea as abnormal respiratory event lasting greater than 10 s with a greater than 30 % reduction in nasal cannula airflow with oxygen desaturation or arousal (Fig. 4.2). Hypopneas are particularly controversial since their definition is broader and this in turn can have significant implications for the final scoring of the PSG. According to AASM criteria hypopnea can be scored using two definitions:

(1) Recommended definition: at least a 30 % reduction in airflow in association with a 3 % oxygen desaturation or arousal.
(2) Acceptable definition: at least a 30 % reduction in airflow in association with a 4 % oxygen desaturation.

Hypopnea can generally be classified as obstructive events if they are associated with snoring or thoraco-abdominal paradoxical breathing.

Table 4.2 SCOPER categorization

Sleep	Cardiovascular	Oximetry	Position	Effort	Respiratory
S_1	**C_1**	**O_1**	**P_1**	**E_1**	**R_1**
Three EEG channels with EOG and chin EMG	>1 ECG lead	Oximetry (finger or ear) with recommended sampling[a]	Video or visual position measurement	Two RIP belts	Nasal pressure and thermal device
S_2	**C_2**	**O_{1x}**	**P_2**	**E_2**	**R_2**
<3 EEGs with or without EOG or chin EMG	Peripheral arterial tonometry	Oximetry (finger or ear) without recommended sampling (per scoring manual) or not described	Nonvisual position measurement	One RIP belt	Nasal pressure
S_3	**C_3**	**O_2**		**E_3**	**R_3**
Sleep surrogate: e.g., actigraphy	Standard ECG measure (one lead)	Oximetry with alternative site (e.g., forehead)		Derived effort	Thermal device
S_4	**C_4**	**O_3**		**E_4**	**R_4**
Other sleep meaures	Derived pulse (typically from oximetry)	Other oximetry		Other effort measures (including piezo belts)	End-tidal CO_2
	C_5				**R_5**
	Other cardiac measures				Other respiratory measures

EEG electroencephalogram, *EOG* electrooculogram, *EMG* electromyogram, *RIP* respiratory inductance plethysmography

[a]Proper oximetry sampling is defined as 3-s averaging and a minimum of 10-Hz sampling rate

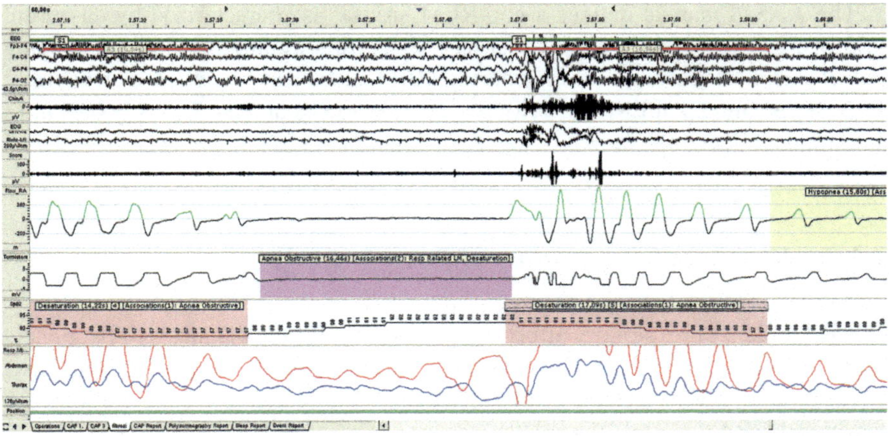

Fig. 4.1 Obstructive apnea

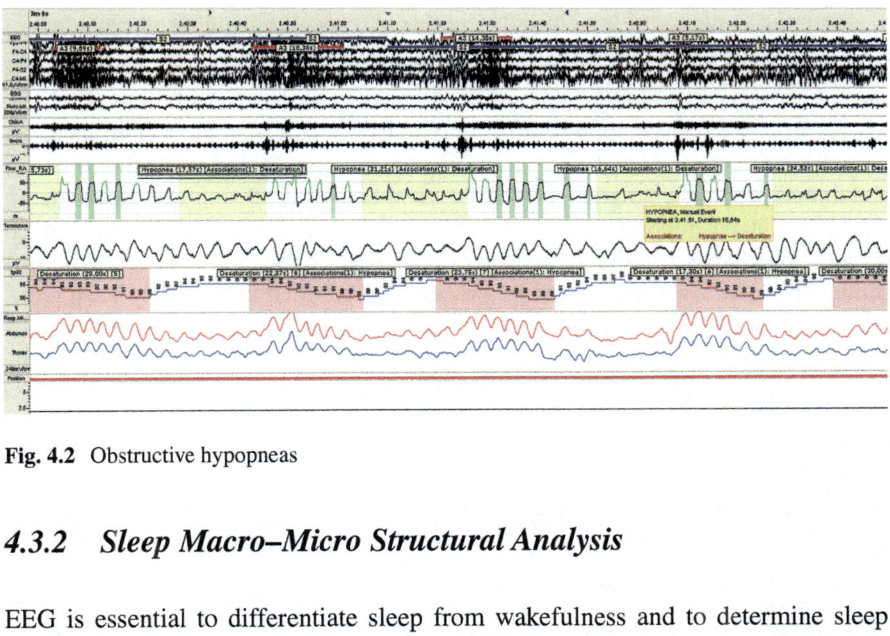

Fig. 4.2 Obstructive hypopneas

4.3.2 Sleep Macro–Micro Structural Analysis

EEG is essential to differentiate sleep from wakefulness and to determine sleep staging [4], and is also essential for the scoring of arousals during sleep. EEG electrodes are placed using the Standard International 10–20 System. EOG is also essential during PSG and records conjugate eye movements in an out-of-phase fashion. Chin EMG is another key component to sleep staging, particularly the scoring of REM sleep. Visual scoring of EEG, EOG and chin EMG data are integrated in order to assign a sleep stage to each 30 s epoch. The manual includes rules for the evaluation of the signals and distinguishes wakefulness, two stages of light sleep, one stage of deep sleep and one stage called REM sleep. Specific rules and definitions of sleep staging are well documented in the AASM scoring manual.

The AASM manual defines a non-REM arousal as characterized by an abrupt shift of EEG frequency lasting for at least 3 s with a minimum of 10 s preceding stable sleep, whereas an arousal during REM sleep also requires a concurrent increase in submental EMG activity for the duration of at least 1 s. Arousals have important clinical implications in the fragmentation of sleep in patients with OSAS.

4.3.3 RERA and Respiratory Effort

The assessment of respiratory effort is a key element for the diagnosis of hypopneic event as obstructive or central, but also is the reference technology for the diagnosis of Respiratory Event Related Arousal (RERA) (Fig. 4.3). The AASM allows for scoring a RERA:

- with a sequence of breaths lasting at least 10 s characterized by increasing respiratory effort or flattening of the nasal pressure waveform leading to an arousal from sleep.
- when the sequence of breaths does not meet criteria for an apnea or hypopnea.

Several methods exist to measure respiratory effort. The most commonly used is respiratory inductive plethysmography (RIP). RIP uses bands with inductive coils placed around the chest and abdomen. RIP detects changes in the electromagnetic properties of the coils and provides a semiquantitative measure of thoracic and abdominal pressure changes. The sum of the thoracic and abdominal signals (sum channel) can be important in identifying paradoxical effort in obstructive sleep apnea. Nevertheless, in the diagnostic clinical routine the sum channel alone is a semiquantitative measure and cannot precisely derive tidal volume, but when properly calibrated the inductance plethysmography signal can provide an estimate of tidal volume [5]. Calibration is uncommon in routine clinical practice due to difficulty maintaining the calibrated signal during changes in body position.

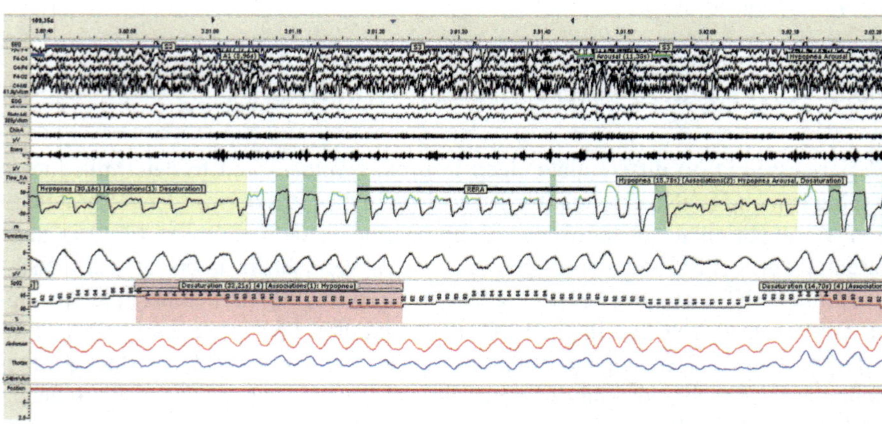

Fig. 4.3 RERA

4.3.4 Gas Exchange Assessment

Finger probe pulse oximetry provides a practical, inexpensive, and noninvasive method of measuring oxygen saturation and is, therefore, the most commonly used technique. Phasic decreases in hemoglobin oxygen saturation of at least 3 % or 4 % are utilized in the current criteria for scoring hypopneas. The accuracy of pulse oximetry in detecting respiratory events can vary depending on the type and averaging time of the oximeter [6]: an averaging time of 3 s or less is suggested [7]. In the absence of airflow limitation, nocturnal oxygen desaturation may suggest other sleep-related breathing disorders, such as obesity hypoventilation syndrome (OHS), neuromyopathy or chronic obstructive pulmonary disease (COPD).

Arterial blood gas (ABG) is the most accurate method and the gold standard for measuring blood oxygenation, but it is invasive, expensive, and impractical for providing continuous monitoring. The associated patient discomfort may adversely affect arousal from sleep. As such, ABG has not gained widespread use in the sleep laboratory setting.

The arterial carbon dioxide partial pressure (Pa CO_2) is considered a reliable marker of alveolar ventilation. Assessing Pa CO_2 is an important component of respiratory monitoring during sleep and without this information it is not possible to advance the diagnosis of alveolar hypoventilation during sleep [1].

The noninvasive most widespread method in clinical routine is the transcutaneous carbon dioxide partial pressure (Pt CO_2) measure, but the method has some limits: it is expensive, it is not easy, and if not properly adjusted Pt CO_2 has the potential to overestimate Pa CO_2. The response time for Pt CO_2 monitoring is slower (50 s) than oximetry (3 s) and that limits its ability to assess ventilation on a breath-to-breath basis.

Another available technology to evaluate Pa CO_2 is the end-tidal carbon dioxide monitoring which involves drawing a stream of air into a chamber and measuring light absorption through the gas chamber. This technique provides an accurate reflection of Pa CO_2 in most patients, although it may underestimate Pa CO_2 in patients with lung diseases (e.g., COPD) and cannot be used with patients on O_2-therapy or noninvasive mechanical ventilation (NIV).

4.3.5 Snoring Recording

The evaluation of sleep-related breathing disorders with PSG generally includes the use of a microphone or piezoelectric sensor to detect snoring. Despite the importance of the symptom, there is currently no widely accepted, validated instrument to quantify snoring for either diagnostic or therapeutic purposes.

4.3.6 Cardiovascular Parameters Recording

Cardiac parameters are assessed by performing a modified ECG. Care must be taken in diagnosing specific cardiac pathology based on a single modified lead [4]. If clinically indicated, a full 12-lead ECG and/or cardiology consultation may be warranted to further evaluate the PSG findings.

4.3.7 Body Position and Limb Movements Recording

A specific sensor can measure body position objectively, however the most reliable assessment of body position is achieved by video monitoring and sleep technician observation. The data from position sensor placed on the chest must be interpreted with caution because the location of the head and neck is often not consistent with that of the chest. Leg movements are measured by two EMG surface electrodes symmetrically placed over each anterior tibialis muscle.

4.3.8 Polysomnographic Report: Indexes and Parameters

Automated scoring of respiratory events using specialized computer software is possible with PSG and portable monitoring devices, but after the preliminary interpretation it is categorically recommended that manual rescoring of the exam be performed by a physician experienced in sleep disorders.

Some indexes and parameters are essential to identify the respiratory sleep disorders (RSD) and define the severity level:

- RDI: apneas + hypopnea + RERA per hour of sleep
- AHI: apneas + hypopnea per hour of sleep
- RDI and AHI in supine position versus non-supine
- ODI : number of phasic desaturation per hour of sleep
- SaO_2 mean: mean saturation during sleep
- CT < 90 %: total sleep time spent with SaO_2 less than 90 %
- Supine time: time spent in supine position

The severity of obstructive sleep apnea is usually graded using the AHI using AASM criteria as follows: mild (>5–15), moderate (>15–30), and severe (>30).

There is also no clear consensus on what AHI cut point defines the presence of clinically significant disease. Studies routinely show a poor correlation between AHI and the severity of patient self-reported symptoms such as excessive daytime sleepiness [8]. Additionally there may be considerable inter-scorer and intra-scorer variability in AHI, and also scoring rules for respiratory events can vary between sleep laboratories, with recent literature showing that use of different hypopnea scoring criteria (i.e., 1999 AASM "Chicago criteria" vs 2007 AASM "recommended" or "alternative" criteria) can result in significant differences in the reported AHI [9]. This confirm the extreme complexity in the interpretation of PSG, which remains the gold standard for diagnosis of OSAS.

4.4 From Standard PSG to Level 3–4 Ambulatory Sleep Testing

The dramatic increase in obesity over the past 30 years, the increasing longevity of the population, and the increasing awareness of OSAS as a risk factor have exponentially increased the number of patients for evaluation. We know from various studies that more than 75 % of patients with OSAS are either undiagnosed or untreated. This is particularly the case among those who are socioeconomically disadvantaged. These phenomena can at least partially explain the growing trend towards ambulatory sleep testing instead of overnight in-lab PSG testing.

When using portable devices the exam is conducted in the patients' own home environment without the need for continuous monitoring by a trained technician. This diagnostic model may have particular relevance for patients in rural and remote regions and in developing countries where health-care resources are limited, however many patients even in first world nations prefer ambulatory sleep testing and feel it is more indicative of their real sleep.

In 2003 the AASM, the American College of Chest Physicians, and the American Thoracic Society published a document that did not support general use of portable monitoring over laboratory PSG due to a lack of sufficient evidence. In 2007, the Portable Monitoring Task Force of the AASM updated clinical guidelines for the use of unattended portable monitors in the diagnosis of OSA. Based on a review of the literature [10] the document recommended that unattended, portable monitoring (recording a minimum of airflow, respiratory effort and oximetry) may be an alternative to PSG for the diagnosis of OSA in patients with a high pretest probability of moderate-to-severe OSA without significant medical comorbidities in conjunction with comprehensive evaluation by a board certified sleep specialist. In 2007 the Centers for Medicare and Medicaid Services in the United States approved the use of a limited home sleep recording device with at least three channels to diagnose OSA for the purposes of reimbursement for CPAP treatment.

A recent survey from Europe demonstrated that ambulatory sleep testing is widely used as an alternative to PSG. Only four out of 22 countries exclusively use full overnight PSG, and in 13 countries ambulatory sleep testing is currently reimbursed [11].

There has also been considerable debate worldwide about the role of portable sleep monitoring in the diagnosis of OSA in particular about the high variability of performances of different monitoring devices, sensitivity and specificity of the exam, applicability of clinical trial results to "real world" populations, and about the uncertainty surrounding the overall cost effectiveness of ambulatory approaches. Several limitations of portable sleep studies need to be considered:

- The potential for signal loss when conducted in an unsupervised setting resulting in increased study failures.
- Since the number of respiratory events are scored per hour of recording (i.e., "respiratory disturbance index") rather than per hour of sleep, the severity of OSA could potentially be under estimated in case of prolonged periods of wakefulness throughout the night. This risk could be mitigated by performing multiple night recordings if the screening technology is cheap enough and can be self-administered.
- The absence of EEG signals limits the ability to score hypopnea.
- There is insufficient literature about the use of portable monitoring level 3–4 on patients with comorbidities (e.g., COPD, neuromyopathies, OHS, heart failure).

There is broad consensus that when a patient provides a clinical history suggestive of sleep disorders other than OSA, such as nocturnal epilepsy, parasomnias, or limb movement disorders, then a standard PSG is needed. In patients who continue to complain of excessive daytime sleepiness despite seemingly adequate treatment of their OSAS, a full PSG may be helpful to identify the presence of other sleep disorders.

4.4.1 Ambulatory Testing Level 3–4 Versus Level 1

The most commonly used ambulatory monitoring devices are type 3 monitors. Noninferiority studies have tried to compare them with in-laboratory PSG for the diagnosis of OSAS. Level 3 portable devices showed good diagnostic performance compared with level 1 sleep tests in adult patients with a high pretest probability of moderate to severe obstructive sleep apnea and no unstable comorbidities [12].

The conclusion demonstrates that the level 3 and 4 monitors are generally accurate to diagnose OSA (as compared to PSG), but have a wide and variable bias in estimating the actual AHI.

References

1. American Academy of Sleep Medicine. International classification of sleep disorders, 3rd ed. American Academy of Sleep Medicine; 2014.
2. Ferber R, Millman R, Coppola M, et al. Portable recording in the assessment of obstructive sleep apnea. Sleep. 1994;17:378–92.
3. Collop NA, Tracy SL, Kapur V, et al. Obstructive sleep apnea devices for out-of-center (OOC) testing: technology evaluation. J Clin Sleep Med. 2011;7:531–48.
4. American Academy of Sleep Medicine. Manual for the scoring of sleep and associated events, version 2.1, 2 July 2014.
5. Whyte KF, Gugger M, Gould GA, et al. Accuracy of respiratory inductive plethysmograph in measuring tidal volume during sleep. J Appl Physiol. 1991;71:1866–71.
6. Zafar S, Ayappa I, Norman RG, et al. Choice of oximeter affects apnea–hypopnea index. Chest. 2005;127:80–8.

7. Farre R, Montserrat JM, Ballester E, et al. Importance of the pulse oximeter averaging time when measuring oxygen desaturation in sleep apnea. Sleep. 1998;21:386–90.
8. Weaver EM, Kapur V, Yueh B. Polysomnography vs self-reported measures in patients with sleep apnea. Arch Otolaryngol Head Neck Surg. 2004;130:453–8.
9. Ruehland WR, Rochford PD, O'Donoghue FJ, et al. The new AASM criteria for scoring hypopneas: impact on the apnea hypopnea index. Sleep. 2009;32:150–7.
10. Collop NA, Anderson WM, Boehlecke B, et al. Clinical guidelines for the use of unattended portable monitors in the diagnosis of obstructive sleep apnea in adult patients. Portable Monitoring Task Force of the American Academy of Sleep Medicine. J Clin Sleep Med. 2007;3:737–47.
11. Fietze I, Penzel T, Alonderis A, et al. Management of obstructive sleep apnea in Europe. Sleep Med. 2011;12(2):190–7. doi:10.1016/j.sleep.2010.10.003 [Epub 2010 Dec 16].
12. El Shayeb M, Topfer LA, Stafinski T, et al. Diagnostic accuracy of level 3 portable sleep tests versus level 1 polysomnography for sleep-disordered breathing: a systematic review and meta-analysis. CMAJ. 2014;186(1):E25–51.

Chapter 5
Imaging

Andrea De Vito, Pier Carlo Frasconi, Oscar Bazzocchi, and Giulia Tenti

5.1 Introduction

Although polysomnography represents the gold standard for the diagnosis of OSA [1], the assessment of upper airway is mandatory in detecting the level, degree, and causes of obstruction, especially if a conservative or surgical treatment has to be appropriately planned. Cephalometry, Computed Tomography (CT), and Magnetic Resonance (MR) are the main imaging modalities applied in the assessment of OSA patients, providing insights into pathophysiology, evaluation, and treatment planning of OSA [2–4]. Two more issues of increasing importance in TORS area are the possibility to detect vessels close to the surgical area in order to prevent inadvertent injury during dissection and the capability from simple linear and angular measures [4] to obtain a sound predictor index about the exposure difficulties in TORS. From the scientific point of view some very interesting studies were published dealing with the volume measurement of the obstructive tissue before surgery, with the comparative measure of the airway volume before and after surgery [5].

In this chapter we review the role of different imaging modalities in the diagnostic assessment of the upper airway in OSA patients, with specific attention to the hypopharynx.

A. De Vito, M.D., Ph.D. (✉) • P.C. Frasconi, M.D.
Head and Neck Department—ENT & Oral Surgery Unit G.B. Morgagni—L. Pierantoni Hospital, Forlì - Infermi Hospital, Faenza - ASL of Romagna, Italy
e-mail: dr.andrea.devito@gmail.com; pfrasco@tin.it

O. Bazzocchi, M.D.
Radiology Unit, G.B. Morgagni—L. Pierantoni Hospital, Forlì, ASL of Romagna, Italy
e-mail: oscar.baz@libero.it

G. Tenti, M.D.
Centro Chirurgico Toscano, Arezzo, Italy
e-mail: giuliatenti@libero.it

© Springer International Publishing Switzerland 2016

C. Vicini et al. (eds.), *TransOral Robotic Surgery for Obstructive Sleep Apnea*,
DOI 10.1007/978-3-319-34040-1_5

5.2 Cephalometry

Cephalometry is a well-standardized analysis of bony and soft tissue structures realized on lateral radiograph of the head and neck region, with the patient in an upright position, which has become one of the standard diagnostic tools in OSA patients. Cephalometry provides measurements of many set points, planes, or distances within the head and neck region, highlighting important differences between normal, snorers, and apneic subjects, especially with regard to the evaluation of skeletal craniofacial morphology. Overall cephalometric studies have shown that specific cephalometric parameters (a retro-position of the maxilla or mandible, a narrow posterior airway space, an enlarged tongue, a thick and long soft palate, and especially an inferiorly located hyoid bone) represent anatomical risk factors for OSA [6–8].

The cephalometric analysis allows the surgeon to obtain anatomically based outcome predictors of surgical treatment, being a standard and mandatory tool for maxillo-facial surgeons in assessing the dento-facial characteristics before and after maxillo-mandibular advancement (MMA) surgery. Moreover preoperative and postoperative cephalometric radiographic analysis after MMA surgery has demonstrated a significant improvement in the posterior airway space caliber, with an increase of pharyngeal volume and a decrease of airway resistance as a consequence [9]. Likewise the cephalometric demonstration of a narrow posterior airway space (PAS $\leq$3.4 mm), a narrow angle from the sella to the nasion and to the supramental point (SNB $<$ 80°), a wider angle from the sella to the nasion and to the subspinal point (SNA $>$ 82°), and a distance between hyoid bone and mandibular plane $>$15 mm was found to have a positive predictive value for mandibular advancement device (MAD) effectiveness in OSA patients [10–12].

Lateral cephalometric radiography represents an accessible, economic, and suitable tool for the evaluation of craniofacial abnormalities in OSA patients, but it is of limited value in the detailed evaluation of soft tissue structures. However, cephalometry allows us to have an effective analysis of the lateral image of the tongue base, its shape in the profile perspective according to the Moore Classification (prevalent upper, diffuse or lower obstruction), its grade of vertical development, and its relation with the pharyngeal posterior wall. The distance between the hyoid bone and mandibular plane (H-MP) represents the most important anatomical landmark to analyze, because it is an indirect measurement of the tongue's vertical height and its role in upper airway collapse, especially when H-MP is greater than 25 mm. In conclusion lateral cephalometry is a low cost tool to provide information about vertical extension of the tongue base which correlates with inferior outcomes if H-MP is greater than 2.5 cm (Fig. 5.1). Furthermore, cephalometry provides two-dimensional static images in the sagittal plane, in awake subjects in an upright position, and it is not possible to realize an accurate analysis of transverse dimensions, cross-sectional shape, or volume of upper airway changes during sleep.

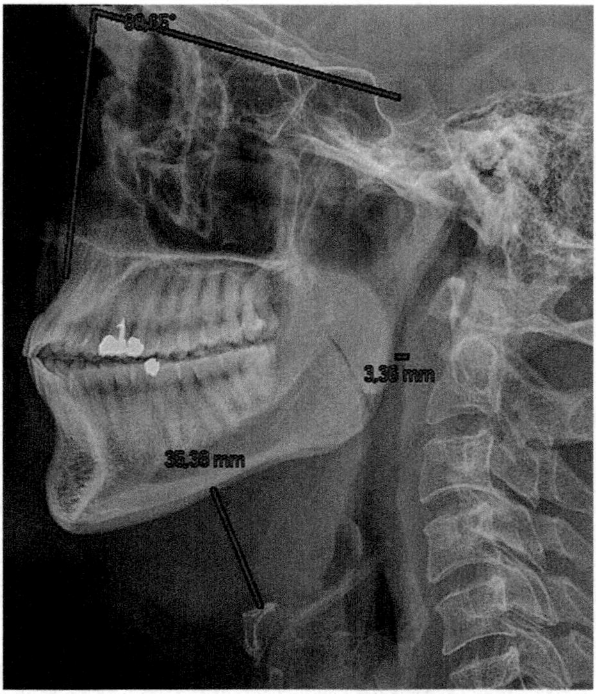

Fig. 5.1 Lateral cephalometry is a low-cost tool to provide information about vertical extension of the tongue base which correlates with inferior outcomes if H-MP is greater than 2.5 cm

5.3 Computed Tomography (CT)

Basic CT techniques applied for the evaluation of the upper airway of OSA patients include standard, axial, and coronal CT images, whereas electron beam CT and helical CT scanners provide dynamic evaluation and volumetric UA images and allow us to analyze the airway dimension during wakefulness and sleep. CT dynamic evaluation of upper airway during states of wakefulness and sleep has shown narrowing predominantly in the retro-palatal region in OSA patients, with a direct relation between the degree of narrowing and OSA severity [13–21].

Volumetric CT studies have shown smaller upper airway diameter and larger tongue volume in obese OSA patients [22, 23], and three-dimensional CT has demonstrated that the most important parameter associated with upper airway obstruction during sleep appears to be the narrowing at the retro-palatal area and narrowing of the lateral airway which correlates with the apnea-hypopnea index (AHI) severity [24].

Three-dimensional multidetector computed tomography (3D MDCT) analysis of the upper airway has also shown that the lengthening of the pharynx may independently contribute to the severity of OSA, in the absence of volumetric change of upper airway soft tissues [25].

A recent study using CT has investigated the relationship between lingual-occlusal surface position and retroglossal obstruction in OSA patients, performing measures of the retroglossal cross-sectional area and inner diameter. The authors have found a significant association between lingual-occlusal surface, retroglossal obstruction, and AHI [26]. CT may also provide more details compared to cephalometry in classifying the tongue base obstruction pattern according to Moore's description, offering the surgeon another predictive tool to improve outcomes.

Although dynamic, volumetric, and three-dimensional CT studies have provided significant insights into OSA pathophysiology, radiation exposure represents a limitation of its application in scientific studies. Likewise, CT scan may have a role in the assessment of the upper airway in the evaluation of OSA patients who are being considered for transoral robotic surgery, especially when the hypopharyngeal endoscopic evaluation shows a predominantly muscular base of the tongue. In this case, computed tomography angiography (CTA) allows us to identify the course of the lingual artery and its branches and provides a safer and more efficient robotic dissection of the base of the tongue [27] (Fig. 5.2). Very recently, a new and very interesting application of CT for TORS was published by [4]: "preoperative measurements of radiographic images of the oropharyngeal working space determined that a distance less than 8 mm from the posterior pharyngeal wall to the soft palate and/or 30 mm from the posterior

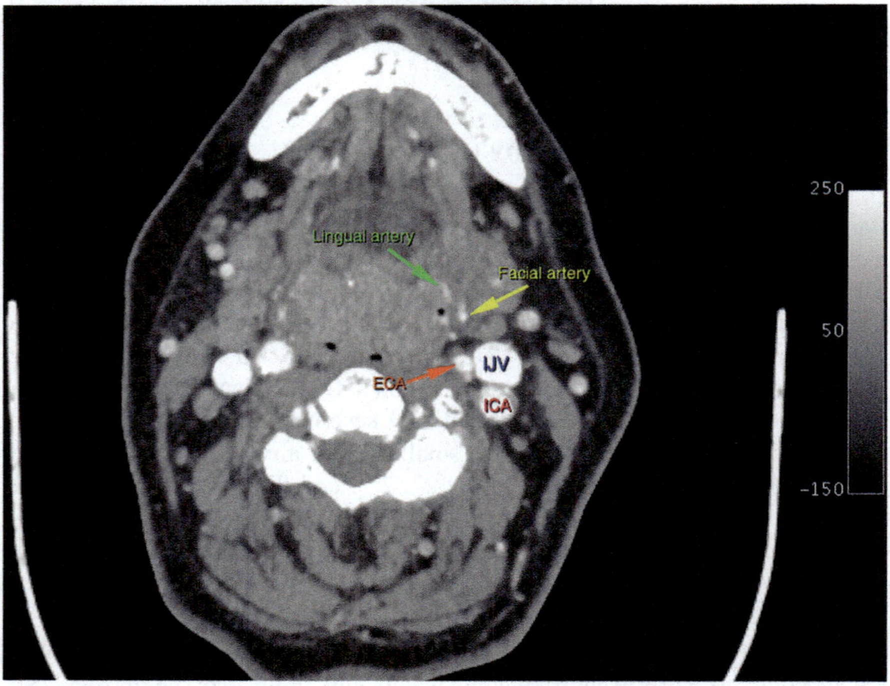

Fig. 5.2 CT allows us to identify the course of the lingual artery and its branches and provides a safer and more efficient robotic dissection of the base of the tongue. *ECA* external carotid artery, *ICA* internal carotid artery; *IJV* internal jugular vein

pharyngeal wall to the hyoid, and/or an angle less than 130° between the epiglottis and larynx, may represent restricted exposure for TORS resection of the tongue base." Bad exposure means less resection and more probable posterior wall damage.

5.4 Magnetic Resonance Imaging (MRI)

MRI represents the best current imaging modality for upper airway evaluation in OSA patients in comparison with lateral cephalometry and CT scan. MRI allows us to achieve an excellent soft tissue contrast, providing precise and accurate measurements of the upper airway and surrounding tissue. MRI basic acquisition includes multiplanar images in axial, sagittal, and coronal planes; likewise volumetric data analysis with three-dimensional reconstructed images is easily obtained.

Overall anatomical MRI studies have shown a statistically significant pharyngeal fat deposition in OSA patients in comparison with healthy controls, especially anterolateral pharyngeal deposition in non-obese OSA patients [28–30]. Volumetric MRI has demonstrated that the volume of soft tissue structures surrounding the upper airway is enlarged in OSA patients, even after controlling for volume of the parapharyngeal fat pads, and that the volume of the tongue and lateral pharyngeal walls were shown to be particularly important as independent risk factors for OSA [31]. MRI also allows a precise definition of lymphoid tissue hypertrophy including location, thickness, and volume ratio between lymphoid tissue and muscle (Fig. 5.3). It allows a better planning of tissue resection before surgery.

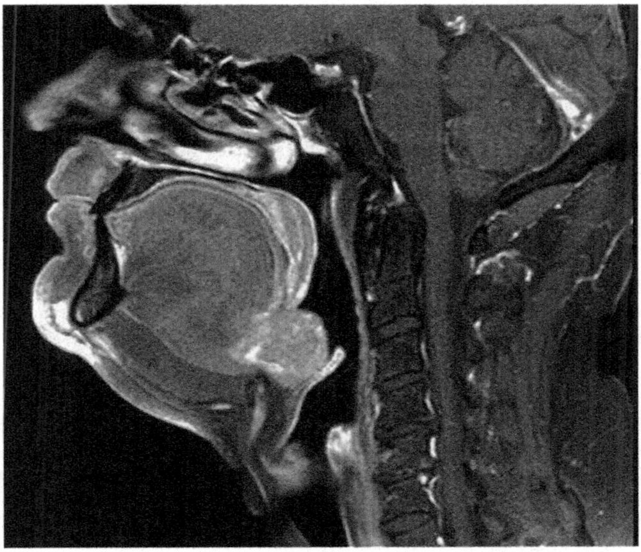

Fig. 5.3 MRI allows a precise definition of lymphoid tissue hypertrophy including location, thickness, and volume ratio between lymphoid tissue and muscle

Furthermore dynamic upper airway assessment obtained by introduction of ultrafast MRI techniques has shown dynamic configuration, motion, and change of the upper airway during normal sleeping and apnea/hypopnea events. During normal sleep, the upper airway remains patent at both the oropharyngeal and retroglossal level with minimal airway motion, whereas during apneic events dynamic MRI clearly shows complete airway collapse at the level of the soft palate and the base of the tongue [32, 33]. In addition dynamic MRI provides unique information about the relationship between tongue base and palate during obstructive events. There are basically two different pathophysiological scenarios: primary and secondary palatal obstruction. Primary palatal obstruction occurs when the soft palate falls back and the tongue base remains stable and does not contribute to posterior displacement of the palate; in this case standalone palate surgery would be enough to correct the obstruction. Secondary palatal obstruction occurs when the palate is pushed back by the tongue base which contributes to the overall obstruction. MRI provides this very important pathophysiological information that would be difficult to obtain by different techniques.

A recent focus of MRI studies in OSA patients is the analysis of the anatomy of the lingual artery and its relation to the adjacent structures. Three-dimensional phase-contrast sequence (3D-PC) of magnetic resonance angiography (MRA) allows us to describe the lingual artery course and its application could be clinically useful before proceeding to transoral robotic surgery, in order to show irregular patterns and prevent intraoperative hemorrhage [34].

Otherwise MRI is still an expensive and not widely available imaging technique; it cannot be performed on patients with pacemakers, difficult to perform in patients with claustrophobia and morbid obesity.

References

1. The Report of an American Academy of Sleep Medicine Task Force. Sleep-related breathing disordered in adults: recommendations for syndrome definition and measurement techniques in clinical research. Sleep. 1999;22:667–89.
2. Goldberg AN, Schwab RJ. Identifying the patient with sleep apnea. Upper airway assessment and physical examination. Otolaryngol Clin North Am. 1998;31(6):919–30.
3. Patel NP, Schwab RJ. Upper airway imaging. In: Kushida CA, editor. Sleep disorders/vol. 4 obstructive sleep apnea. Diagnosis and treatment; 2007. Chapter 4. p. 61–88.
4. Luginbuhl A, Baker A, Curry J, Drejet S, Miller M, Cognetti D. Preoperative cephalometric analysis to predict transoral robotic surgery exposure. J Robot Surg. 2014;8(4):313–7 [Epub 2014 Jun 24].
5. Chiffer RC, Schwab RJ, Keenan BT, Borek RC, Thaler ER. Volumetric MRI analysis pre- and post-transoral robotic surgery for obstructive sleep apnea. Laryngoscope. 2015;125(8):1988–95.
6. Ryu HH, Kim CH, Cheon SM, et al. The usefulness of cephalometric measurement as a diagnostic tool for obstructive sleep apnea syndrome: a retrospective study. Oral Surg Oral Med Oral Pathol Oral Radiol. 2015;119(1):20–31.
7. Shepard JW, Gefter WB, Guilleminault C, et al. Evaluation of the upper airway in patients with obstructive sleep apnea. Sleep. 1991;14(4):361–71.
8. Nelson S, Hans M. Contribution of craniofacial risk factors in increasing apneic activity among obese and non-obese habitual snorers. Chest. 1997;111(1):154–62.

9. Waite PD, Vilos GA. Surgical changes of posterior airway space in obstructive sleep apnea. Oral Maxillofac Surg Clin North Am. 2002;14:385–99.
10. Guarda-Nardini L, Manfredini D, Mion M, et al. Anatomically based outcome predictors of treatment for obstructive sleep apnea with intraoral splint devices: a systematic review of cephalometric studies. J Clin Sleep Med. 2015; Apr 10.
11. Horiuchi A, Suzuki M, Ookubo M, et al. Measurement techniques predicting the effectiveness of an oral appliance for obstructive sleep apnea hypopnea syndrome. Angle Orthod. 2005;75:1003–11.
12. Skinner MA, Robertson CJ, Kingshott RN, et al. The efficacy of mandibular advancement splint in relation to cephalometric variables. Sleep Breath. 2002;63:315–24.
13. Aksoz T, Akan H, Celebi M, Sakan BB. Does the oropharyngeal fat tissue influence the oropharyngeal airway in snorers? Dynamic CT study. Korean J Radiol. 2004;5(2):102–6.
14. Akan H, Aksoz T, Belet U, Sesen T. Dynamic upper airway soft-tissue and caliber changes in healthy subjects and snoring patients. AJNR Am J Neuroradiol. 2004;25(10):1846–50.
15. Burger CD, Stanson AW, Daniels BK, Sheedy II PF, Shepard Jr JW. Fast-CT evaluation of the effect of lung volume on upper airway size and function in normal men. Am Rev Respir Dis. 1992;146(2):335–9.
16. Burger CD, Stanson AW, Sheedy II PF, Daniels BK, Shepard Jr JW. Fast-computed tomography evaluation of age-related changes in upper airway structure and function in normal men. Am Rev Respir Dis. 1992;145(4 Pt 1):846–52.
17. Caballero P, Alvarez-Sala R, Garcia-Rio F, et al. CT in the evaluation of the upper airway in healthy subjects and in patients with obstructive sleep apnea syndrome. Chest. 1998;113(1):111–6.
18. Ell SR, Jolles H, Galvin JR. Cine CT demonstration of nonfixed upper airway obstruction. AJR Am J Roentgenol. 1986;146(4):669–77.
19. Ell SR, Jolles H, Keyes WD, Galvin JR. Cine CT technique for dynamic airway studies. AJR Am J Roentgenol. 1985;145(1):35–6.
20. Galvin JR, Rooholamini SA, Stanford W. Obstructive sleep apnea: diagnosis with ultrafast CT. Radiology. 1989;171(3):775–8.
21. Haponik EF, Smith PL, Bohlman ME, Allen RP, Goldman SM, Bleecker ER. Computerized tomography in obstructive sleep apnea. Correlation of airway size with physiology during sleep and wakefulness. Am Rev Respir Dis. 1983;127(2):221–6.
22. Fleetham JA. Upper airway imaging in relation to obstructive sleep apnea. Clin Chest Med. 1992;13(3):399–416.
23. Ryan CF, Lowe AA, Li D, Fleetham JA. Three-dimensional upper airway computed tomography in obstructive sleep apnea. A prospective study in patients treated by uvulopalatopharyngoplasty. Am Rev Respir Dis. 1991;144(2):428–32.
24. Li HY, Chen NH, Wang CR, Shu YH, et al. Use of 3-dimensional computed tomography scan to evaluate upper airway patency for patients undergoing sleep-disordered breathing surgery. Otolaryngol Head Neck Surg. 2003;129(4):336–42.
25. Kim EJ, Choi JH, Kim YS, et al. Upper airway changes in severe obstructive sleep apnea: upper airway length and volumetric analyses using 3D MDCT. Acta Otolaryngol. 2011;131(5):527–32.
26. Li S1, Qin Y, Wu D. Lingual-occlusal surface position predicts retroglossal obstruction in patients with obstructive sleep apnea hypopnea syndrome. Acta Otolaryngol. 2015; June 24:1–6 [Epub ahead of print].
27. Wu D, Qin J, Guo X, et al. Analysis of the difference in the course of the lingual arteries caused by tongue position change. Laryngoscope. 2015;125(3):762–6.
28. Mortimore IL, Marshall I, Wraith PK. Neck and total body fat deposition in nonobese and obese patients with sleep apnea compared with that in control subjects. Am J Respir Crit Care Med. 1998;157:280–3.
29. Sittitavornwong S, Waite PD. Imaging the upper airway in patients with sleep disordered breathing. Oral Maxillofac Surg Clin North Am. 2009;21:389–402.

30. Razek AAKA. Diagnostic role of magnetic resonance imaging in obstructive sleep apnea syndrome. J Comput Assist Tomogr. 2015;39(4):565–71.
31. Schwab RJ, Pasirstein M, Pierson R, et al. Identification of upper airway anatomic risk factors for obstructive sleep apnea with volumetric magnetic resonance imaging. Am J Respir Crit Care Med. 2003;168(5):522–30.
32. Ciscar MA, Juan G, Martinez V, et al. Magnetic resonance imaging of the pharynx in OSA patients and healthy subjects. Eur Respir J. 2001;17(1):79–86.
33. Schwab RJ. Upper airway imaging. Clin Chest Med. 1998;19(1):33–54.
34. Kami YN, Chikui T, Shiraushi T, et al. A new method for displaying the lingual artery using high-resolution three-dimensional phase-contrast magnetic resonance angiography. IJOM. 2013;42(11):1494–8.

Chapter 6
Drug-Induced Sedation Endoscopy (DISE)

Aldo Campanini, Bhik Kotecha, and Erica R. Thaler

6.1 Introduction

Polysomnography (PSG) is the gold standard for functional diagnosis of OSA (number of obstructive events per hour) [1], but it cannot provide detailed anatomic localization of the obstructive sites (anatomical diagnosis).

Drug-induced sedation/sedated or sleep endoscopy (DISE) is a fiber-optic examination of the upper airway under controlled sedation to determine the exact site(s) of upper airway collapse in patients with sleep-disordered breathing.

Quantifying the location and mechanism of upper airway collapse with DISE in an apneic patient can potentially be used to tailor surgical treatments and improve surgical outcomes.

In 1991 Croft and Pringle [2] described an original way to study OSA patients, by "sleep nasendoscopy," a procedure designed to observe the upper airway under pharmacologically induced sleep. The technique however has been labelled with controversies, which have been subsequently and adequately addressed. The main criticism

A. Campanini, M.D. (✉)
Head and Neck Department—ENT & Oral Surgery Unit, G.B. Morgagni—L. Pierantoni Hospital, ASL of Romagna, Forlì, Italy

Infermi Hospital, ASL of Romagna, Faenza, Italy
e-mail: aldocampanini@alice.it

B. Kotecha, M.B.B.Ch., M.Phil., F.R.C.S.
Royal National Throat, Nose & Ear Hospital, 330 Grays Inn Road, London, UK

E.R. Thaler, M.D., F.A.C.S.
Division of General Otolaryngology, Head and Neck Surgery, Department of Otolaryngology-Head and Neck Surgery, University of Pennsylvania School of Medicine, Philadelphia, PA, USA

© Springer International Publishing Switzerland 2016

C. Vicini et al. (eds.), *TransOral Robotic Surgery for Obstructive Sleep Apnea*,
DOI 10.1007/978-3-319-34040-1_6

would seem to be that natural physiological sleep is different from sleep induced during DISE. Numerous studies have subsequently looked at sleep architecture during sedation to demonstrate similarities. The depth of sedation was questioned as differing degrees of obstruction would be observed depending on how deep the sedation was. This was rectified by utilizing bispectral index monitoring (BIS®, Medtronic, Minneapolis, MN, USA) instead of simple clinical judgment (patient's capability to react to different verbal and tactile stimuli). Inter- and intra-observation variations may exist and studies have demonstrated good correlation. This has become of increasing interest in the medical community, as evidenced by the increasing number of articles concerning its use and by its ever-increasing practice worldwide.

In 2014, a European Position Paper [3] defined DISE as drug-induced sedation endoscopy instead of drug-induced sleep endoscopy, considered more appropriate to define the pharmacological condition as "sedation" instead of "sleep." In keeping with this distinction, we have titled our chapter in the same manner. A recent comprehensive of the literature by Ravesloot and De Vries [4] in patients undergoing DISE indicated that collapse occurs in different upper airway regions, including the velopharynx, oropharynx, tongue base, and epiglottis, and that multilevel collapse was often observed.

6.2 The UK Experience

DISE was introduced at our institute and to date more than 7000 procedures have been performed with published data of 2485 patients reported in a retrospective audit [5]. We have continued to use the original Croft and Pringle classification with minor modifications. We have experimented with various sedative agents and our current preference is to use a combination of Midazolam® and Propofol®. We use BIS® monitoring to attain an appropriate level of sedation.

Patients undergoing TORS surgery would typically have moderate or severe OSA and would have previously tried and failed CPAP therapy or oral appliances. All of these patients would undergo DISE and most would demonstrate either Croft and Pringle grade 3- or 5-type findings. Some may have had palatal and oropharyngeal surgery and the grade 5 patients would be suitable for TORS hypopharyngeal surgery.

6.3 The US Experience

When considering multilevel surgery to manage patients with OSA who are CPAP failures, it is imperative to have an anatomic assessment of the locations of collapse. This has been well demonstrated in the literature. For example, using DISE, Kezirian showed that patients who failed upper airway surgery had residual upper airway collapse in the palatal region and/or coexisting hypopharyngeal collapse [6]. Various subjective methods and scoring systems (NOHL, VOTE) [7, 8] have been utilized to help guide the surgeon in determining when and where surgery is appropriate, but none has been definitively correlated with surgical outcome. We have attempted to use a quantitative measurement to further assess DISE patterns of collapse.

6.3.1 Penn DISE Protocol

Our patients are CPAP noncompliant and are interested in pursuing surgery for the management of their OSA. DISE is not performed on patients in whom only palatal/tonsil surgery is deemed sufficient for control of OSA. Any patient being considered for TORS must have DISE as part of their preoperative assessment.

Our patients undergo Propofol®-induced DISE in the operating room, with standard monitoring and resuscitation equipment present. Patients are positioned supine with a standard head cradle to maintain neutral position. No topical anesthetics are used for the nasal or pharyngeal mucosa, nor are any drying agents, such as glycopyrrolate, used. The Propofol® infusion rate is performed in the manner described by Mandel [9]. Propofol® concentrations are determined by modeling using total body mass and age to predict effect site concentration, causing a steady increase in effect over 6 min. Mandel's method allows for a near-constant increment in probability of loss of consciousness (Fig. 6.1). We define wakefulness as the period during which

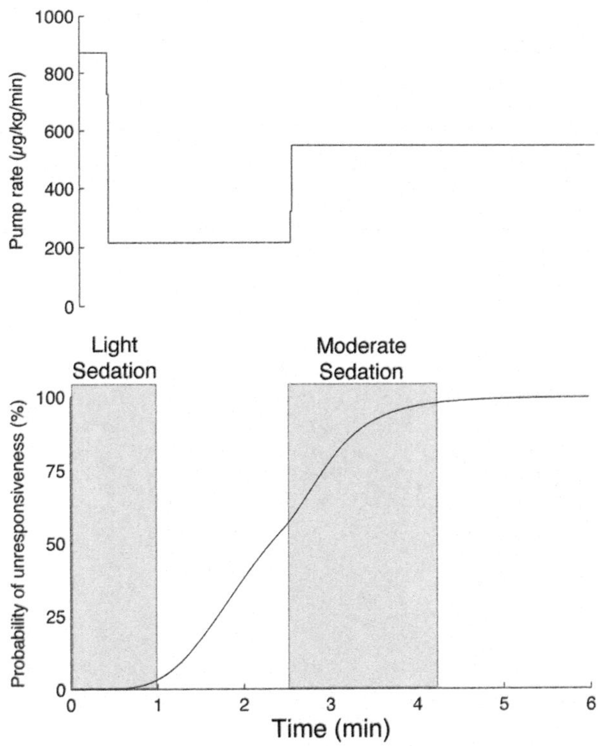

Fig. 6.1 Representation of the Propofol infusion concentrations and sedation state over time in a single patient. The *top panel* demonstrates an infusion sequence leading to an associated effect site concentration and a near-constant increment in the probability of loss of responsiveness (*bottom panel*)

the patient is under light sedation (effect site concentration less than 1 μg/ml), and sleep as the period during which the patient is under moderate sedation (effect site concentration of 2.94 ± .97 μg/ml) (Fig. 6.2).

We use a pediatric bronchoscope for visualization and make measurements at three levels: the velopharynx or retropalatal (RP) region, the hypopharynx or retroglossal (RG) region, and retroepiglottic (RE) region. These three areas are assessed during light and deep sedation, with still photographs and video obtained of each site during both phases.

We then perform image analysis of the three locations using Amira 4.2.1 by Visage Imaging® (Richmond, Victoria, Australia), taking linear measurements in the lateral and anterior-posterior direction as well as cross-sectional area [10]. We have begun to assess the ability of these objective measurements to allow for prediction of surgical success in TORS for OSA, but do not have the N requisite to reach any statistically significant conclusions.

6.4 Italian Experience

6.4.1 Case Series

Our DISE experience as a diagnostic tool *in selected patients* with sleep-disordered breathing (SDB) started in November 2005, but DISE for TORS was born a few years later. In May 2008 we performed our first tongue base resection (TBR) by TORS in a patient with extreme tongue base lymphatic hypertrophy causing isolated retrolingual obstruction.

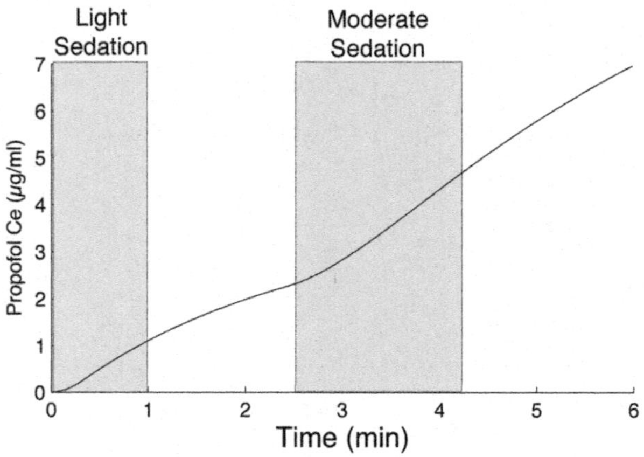

Fig. 6.2 Representation of the Propofol concentration and sedation state over time in a single patient. The *shaded regions* represent the time periods associated with the wake (light sedation) and sleep (moderate sedation) periods during which the wake and sleep images were extracted from the endoscopy video

Our policy is to perform DISE on *all patients* who are potential candidates for TORS treatment.

To date, we have performed about 1000 DISE for OSA; we have completed 222 TORS cases, all of whom received preoperative DISE. It is notable that after our clinical and radiological pre-selection for TORS 25 % of the cases were eliminated because the DISE findings did not fit into our selection criteria for TORS including lateral or circumferential collapse or exclusive palate collapse.

6.4.2 Forlì's DISE Protocol

We started DISE in November 2005 in selected patients, using Propofol® (by bolus technique and then by infusion pump) with an anesthesiologist in the operating room. Since 2009 we have been following the same basic protocol as published in 2010 [11] and according to the options recently validated in the European Position Paper on DISE [3], that is:

- *Patient selection for DISE*:
  - PSG findings do not match awake endoscopic findings (sleep studies/awake endoscopic mismatch)
  - TORS work-up
  - Suspected isolated supraglottic obstruction
  - Surgical failures
  - Suspected stridor related to multisystemic atrophy
- *Setting*:
  - Operating room
  - ENT and anesthesia team
  - No topical decongestion or topical anesthesia
  - No systemic drying agent (atropine, glycopyrrolate)
  - Quiet and darkroom
- *Technical equipment*:
  - Standard monitoring (SaO_2, ECG, blood pressure)
  - TCI® (Target Control Infusion)—not available in the USA
  - Bispectral (BIS®) index
  - Video and audio recording
  - Simultaneous cardiorespiratory monitoring in selected cases (e.g., Embletta®)
- *Patient positioning and diagnostic maneuvers*:
  - Standard supine primary position (with or without pillow)
  - Trans-nasal fiber-optic endoscopy (in selected cases trans-oral also)
  - Mandibular advancement, mouth open/close comparison
- *Drug*: Propofol®

- *Observation window*:
  - At least two or more cycles (snoring, collapse) for each segment of the upper airway
  - Cycle definition: a complete and stable sequence of snoring—obstructing hypo/apnea—oxygen desaturation—breathing
  - BIS® level around 60 or desaturation level close to the previously registered lowest O_2 saturation at the sleep study
- *Target events*:
  - Snoring: pharyngeal and/or laryngeal vibration
  - Apnea–hypopnea: partial or complete pharyngeal obstruction and collapse pattern (lateral, anteroposterior, circumferential)
  - Epiglottic trap-door phenomenon or different patterns of collapse
  - Laryngeal stridor
- *Classification system*:
  - NOHL classification system as described [7]
- *Contraindications*:
  - *Absolute*: ASA 4, pregnancy, allergy to Propofol®
  - *Relative*: morbid obesity

6.4.3 DISE Why?

In 2010 we published [12] a retrospective study on 250 consecutive patients making a comparison between awake and DISE findings. In this study, we found significant differences between hypopharyngeal *degree* and *pattern* of obstruction (59 % and 49 %, respectively) and we discovered that up to 30 % of cases demonstrated laryngeal obstruction by DISE; it was classified as primary if the collapse was produced by intrinsic instability of the larynx or secondary if the tongue base or the lateral wall was responsible for the supraglottic collapse. Endoscopic findings are essential to guide the surgical decision making. It has to be acknowledged that awake endoscopy may frequently underestimate the degree of the hypopharyngeal and laryngeal obstruction.

As we observed in the larynx, we have seen retropalatal obstruction during DISE that may be primary or secondary.

6.4.4 DISE and TORS Failures

We carried out a retrospective unpublished study on 180 patients (83 % males) comparing pre-op DISE findings and success rate after surgery (TORS or multilevel surgery including TORS). Pre-op data (age, AHI, BMI, ESS, and cumulative NOHL score) are described in Table 6.1. DISE cumulative NOHL score seems to be a good index, because linear regression shows a direct correlation between NOHL score versus AHI and versus BMI (Figs. 6.3 and 6.4). The volume of tongue base tissue removed by TORS (180 pts) was 12.0 ± 4.6 (range 3–33 ml). Palatal surgery was performed in 68 % of patients (UPPP 22 %, expansion sphincter pharyngoplasty 46 %) as part of multilevel surgery including TORS.

In order to evaluate DISE staging system as predictor of success, we stated as success criteria post-op AHI <20 and reduction >50 %. The multivariate logistic analysis showed that hypopharyngeal and laryngeal obstructions are significant predictors of success (Fig. 6.5), and the most favorable predictor of success was the anteroposterior pattern of collapse (odds ratio 3.1) (Fig. 6.6).

Table 6.1 Pre-op data (age, AHI, BMI, ESS, and cumulative NOHL score) of 180 patients underwent TORS or multilevel surgery including TORS (unpublished data)

	Min	Max	Mean	SD
Age	16	81	50.3	10.9
Pre-op BMI	22	38.5	28.1	3.6
Pre-op AHI	8.3	98.8	42.3	19.6
Pre-op ESS	0	24	12.0	5.1
Pre-op cumulative NOHL score	5	12	9.9	1.3

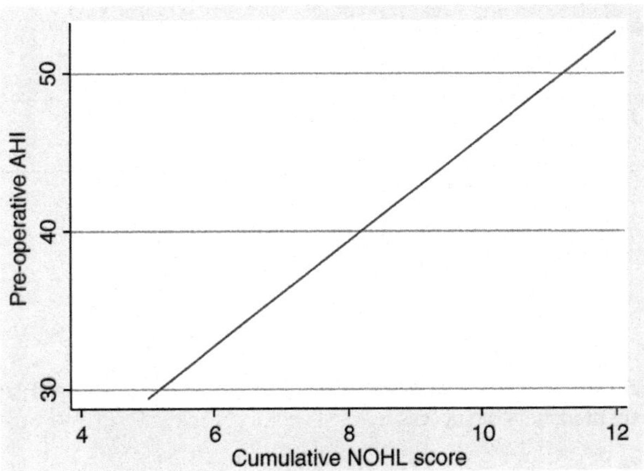

Fig. 6.3 DISE cumulative NOHL score seems to be a good index because linear regression shows a direct correlation between NOHL score and AHI

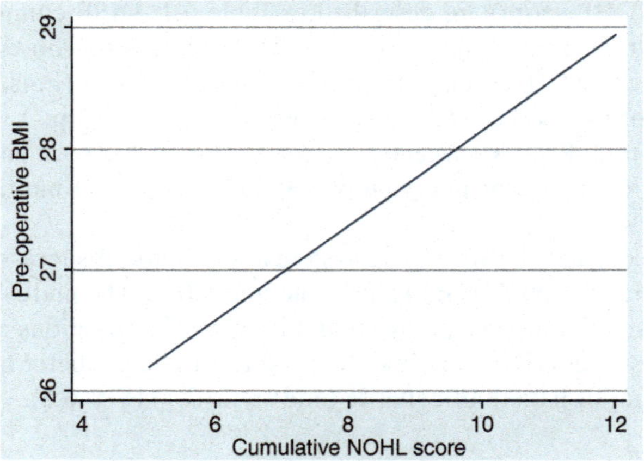

Fig. 6.4 DISE cumulative NOHL score seems to be a good index, because linear regression shows a direct correlation between NOHL score and BMI

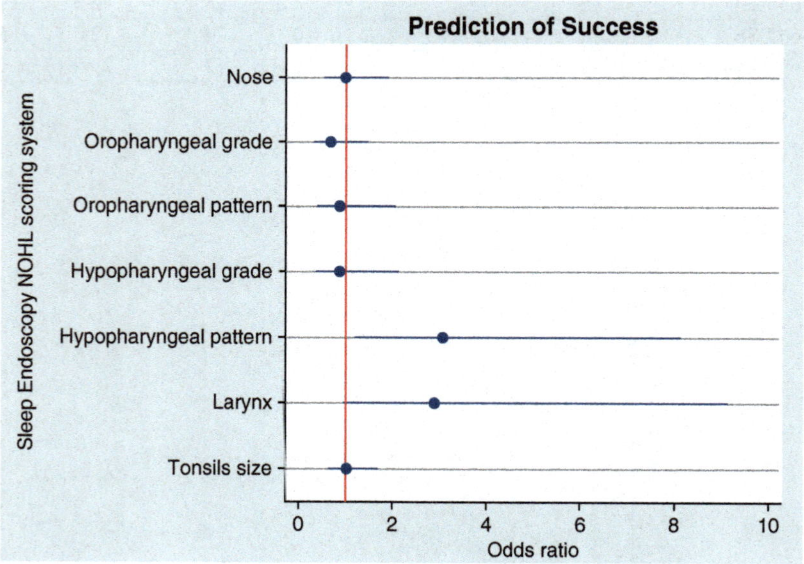

Fig. 6.5 The multivariate logistic analysis showed that hypopharyngeal and laryngeal obstructions are significant predictors of success

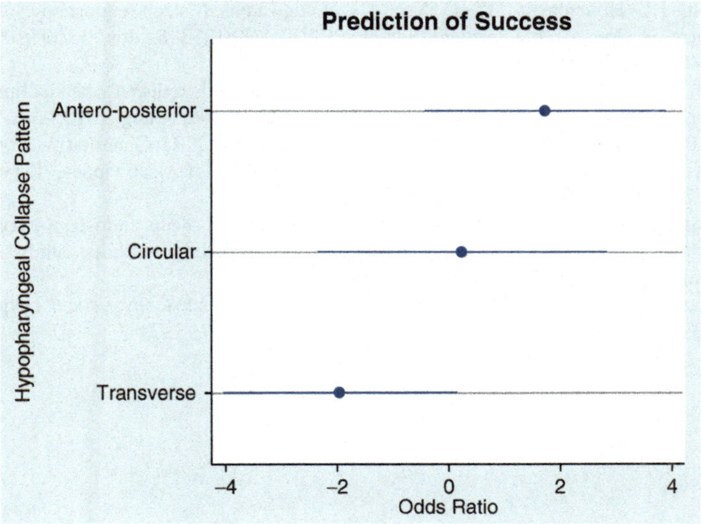

Fig. 6.6 The multivariate logistic analysis showed that the most favorable predictor of success was the anteroposterior pattern of collapse (odds ratio 3.1)

6.5 Conclusion

For successful surgical outcomes, accurate upper airway evaluation and careful patient selection are mandatory. Perhaps an ideal technique for evaluating upper airway obstruction does not exist. DISE, however, remains one of the best tools for evaluating upper airway obstructions for those patients considering surgical intervention.

References

1. Kushida CA, Littner MR, Morgenthaler T, et al. Practice parameters for the indications for *polysomnography* and related procedures: an update for 2005. Sleep. 2005;28:499–521.
2. Croft CB, Pringle M. Sleep nasendoscopy: a technique of assessment in snoring and obstructive sleep apnoea. Clin Otolaryngol Allied Sci. 1991;16:504–9.
3. De Vito A, Carrasco Llatas M, Agnoletti V, et al. European position paper on drug-induced sedation endoscopy (DISE). Sleep Breath. 2014;18(3):453–65.
4. Ravesloot MJL, de Vries N. One hundred consecutive patients undergoing drug-induced sleep endoscopy: results and evaluation. Laryngoscope. 2011;121:2710–6.
5. Kotecha BT, Hannan AS, Khalil HMB, et al. Sleep nasendoscopy: a 10 year retrospective audit study. Eur Arch Otorhinolaryngol. 2007;264:1361–7.
6. Kezirian EJ. Nonresponders to pharyngeal surgery for obstructive sleep apnea: insights from drug-induced sleep endoscopy. Laryngoscope. 2011;121(6):1320–6.
7. Vicini C, De Vito A, Benazzo M, Frassineti S, Campanini A, Frasconi P, Mira E. The nose oropharynx hypopharynx and larynx (NOHL) classification: a new system of diagnostic standardized examination for OSAHS patients. Eur Arch Otorhinolaryngol. 2012;269(4):1297–300.

8. Kezirian EJ, Hohenhorst W, de Vries N. Drug-induced sleep endoscopy: the VOTE classification. Eur Arch Otorhinolaryngol. 2011;268(8):1233–6. doi:10.1007/s00405-011-1633-8 [Epub 2011 May 26].
9. Mandel JE, Sarraf E. The variability of response to propofol is reduced when a clinical observation is incorporated in the control: a simulation study. Anesth Analg. 2012;114(6):1221–9.
10. Borek RC, Thaler ER, Kim C, Jackson N, Mandel JE, Schwab RJ. Quantitative airway analysis during drug-induced sleep endoscopy for evaluation of sleep apnea. Laryngoscope. 2012;122(11):2592–9.
11. De Vito A, Agnoletti V, Berrettini S, et al. Drug-induced sleep endoscopy: conventional versus target controlled infusion techniques—a randomized controlled study. Eur Arch Otorhinolaryngol. 2011;268(3):457–62.
12. Campanini A, Canzi P, De Vito A, et al. Awake versus sleep endoscopy: personal experience in 250 OSAHS patients. Acta Otorhinolaryngol Ital. 2010;30(2):73–7.

Chapter 7
Patient Selection

Tiffany Ann Glazer, Paul T. Hoff, Matthew E. Spector, Claudio Vicini, Filippo Montevecchi, Neil S. Tolley, and Asit Arora

7.1 Introduction

Obstructive sleep apnea hypopnea syndrome (OSAHS) is a significant worldwide health care problem, given the well-known association of OSAHS to cardiopulmonary and neurologic sequela. The surgical management of OSAHS is appealing to both patients and providers as a single intervention that could limit health care costs and avoid the use of continuous positive airway pressure (CPAP). While CPAP is an extremely effective in the treatment of OSAHS, its tolerability, adherence to its use, and the social stigma make it difficult for many patients. Despite multiple available procedures to surgically treat OSAHS, current treatments continue to rely on careful patient selection and appropriate application of surgical interventions. The purpose of this chapter is to discuss appropriate patient selection when considering transoral robotic surgery (TORS) as surgical treatment of OSAHS.

T.A. Glazer, M.D. • P.T. Hoff, M.S., M.D. (✉) • M.E. Spector, M.D.
Department of Otolaryngology—Head and Neck Surgery, University of Michigan Health System, Ann Arbor, MI, USA
e-mail: tglazer@med.umich.edu; phoff@med.umich.edu; mspector@med.umich.edu

C. Vicini, M.D. • F. Montevecchi, M.D.
Head and Neck Department - ENT & Oral Surgery Unit - G.B. Morgagni - L. Pierantoni Hospital, Forlì – Infermi Hospital, Faenza - ASL of Romagna, Italy

N.S. Tolley, M.D., F.R.C.S., D.L.O. • A. Arora, Ph.D., M.R.C.S., D.O.H.N.S.
Department of Otorhinolaryngology and Head & Neck Surgery, St. Mary's Hospital, Imperial College Healthcare NHS Trust, London, UK
e-mail: N.Tolley@imperial.ac.uk

© Springer International Publishing Switzerland 2016

C. Vicini et al. (eds.), *TransOral Robotic Surgery for Obstructive Sleep Apnea*,
DOI 10.1007/978-3-319-34040-1_7

7.2 Optimization of Comorbidities

The preoperative and perioperative management of patients with OSAHS is challenging, as often these patients will have coexisting illnesses such as systemic hypertension, systolic and diastolic myocardial dysfunction, insulin resistance, pulmonary hypertension, stroke, coronary artery disease, and cardiac arrhythmias. Several studies have described perioperative complications associated with OSAHS which include higher reintubation rates, hypercapnia, oxygen desaturations, cardiac arrhythmias, myocardial injury, delirium, unplanned ICU transfers, and longer hospitalization stays [1, 2]. Moreover, the administration of anesthesia exacerbates the upper airway anatomic alterations that lead to pharyngeal collapse in patients with OSAHS. Therefore, appropriate measures should be taken to identify and treat patients with OSAHS and comorbidities to reduce their perioperative risk. Patients with a lower American Society of Anesthesiologists (ASA) score, which measures a patient's systemic fitness before surgery, less than three have been found to have greater success with TORS for OSAHS [3].

Preoperative management should begin with a detailed history of physical exam with emphasis on airway examination as mask ventilation and tracheal intubation are often more difficult in patients with OSAHS [4]. Comorbidities such as hypertension, diabetes mellitus, and congestive heart failure should be assessed for adequacy of control. Any patient with uncontrolled hypertension, hyperglycemia, or decompensated heart failure should be referred to his or her primary care physician for medical optimization prior to surgery [2].

7.3 Polysomnography

The gold standard for the diagnosis of OSAHS is polysomnography (PSG). A variety of sleep studies are available, including Type 1 attended PSG in which multiple measurements are collected including EEG, ECG, EMG, oxygen saturation, airflow monitoring, chest movement, blood pressure, and positioning during sleep. Type 2 studies are unattended and measure at least seven of these parameters. Type 3 and 4 studies are unattended and measure a minimum of 4 and 3 channels, respectively. There are portable (Type 2–4) monitoring systems available and these are used in countries such as Italy, where formal PSG is reserved for selected patients (5 %). The sleep study report includes the apnea/hypopnea index (AHI), or the number of apneas and hypopneas that occur per hour. Other factors include sleep latency, duration, efficiency, and snoring. The respiratory disturbance index (RDI) includes all events (not only apneas and hypopneas) that occur per hour. Taken together, the PSG defines the severity of OSAHS and can help guide the clinician to identify patients who may be successful with surgical interventions [5].

Mild OSAHS is defined as 5–14 AHI events per hour, moderate OSAHS with 15–29 AHI events per hour, and severe OSAHS with ≥30 AHI events per hour. Patients with moderate to severe OSAHS (AHI>20) are potential candidates for TORS; patients with mild to moderate OSAHS (AHI 5–15 and 16–30) may be amenable to other treatments including oral appliance or tonsillectomy and uvulopalatopharyngoplasty/lateral expansion pharyngoplasty with or without thyro-hyoidopexy [5, 6].

In a review of 121 patients who underwent TORS ± multilevel surgery for OSAHS, it was found that patients with severe OSAHS had more improvement, success, and cure 3 months after surgery than their moderate counterparts (Table 7.1) [3].

7.4 Subjective Measurements

Subjective measurements of sleepiness and snoring have been developed and are commonly used as a measure of treatment success. The Epworth sleepiness scale is a 24-point scale measuring subjective sleepiness in eight different scenarios. The Thornton snoring scale is a similar scale in which the patient evaluates the effect of disruptive snoring on his or her relationship in different scenarios. Both should be measured before and after surgery. More comprehensive measures of quality of life include the functional outcome of sleepiness questionnaire (FOSQ) and the shortened FOSQ—10. These questionnaires have been validated and are easy to administer.

A careful assessment of preoperative swallowing function should be performed. The Dysphagia handicap index or the MD Anderson Dysphagia Index will help to avoid the mistake of performing tongue base surgery on patients with underlying pathology that affects swallowing function—most commonly due to advanced age. Documentation of preoperative and postoperative swallowing is important particularly if dysphagia is due to obstructing lingual tonsils.

Table 7.1 A retrospective review of 121 patients who underwent transoral robotic surgery (TORS) ± multilevel surgery for obstructive sleep apnea hypopnea syndrome (OSAHS). Improvement was defined as any decrease in preoperative apnea hypopnea index (AHI). Success was defined as both AHI < 20 and decrease by 50 %. Cure was defined as AHI < 5. In general, patients with severe OSAHS (defined as AHI ≥ 30) achieved greater improvement, success, and cure rates than those with moderate OSAHS (AHI 15–29) [3]

	Moderate OSAHS	Severe OSAHS
Improvement	79.5 % (31/39)	86.6 % (71/82)
Success	48.7 % (19/39)	52.4 % (43/82)
Cure	7.7 % (3/39)	17.1 % (14/82)

7.5 Physical Exam Findings (Table 7.2)

7.5.1 Nasal Examination

In-office physical examination of the upper airway is essential to successful TORS. Severe nasal obstruction due to septal deformity may preclude transnasal intubation. Any nasal deformity including deviated septum, inferior turbinate hypertrophy, adenoid hypertrophy should be addressed at the time of drug induced sleep endoscopy (DISE), which is discussed in detail in Chap. 6. Radiofrequency ablation of the inferior turbinates can be done as an in-office procedure or added to DISE without the need for general anesthesia [5].

7.5.2 Examination for Access

Not all patients are suitable candidates for TORS. Appropriate exposure of the target region is a key factor. The target region will invariably be difficult to remove if its boundaries are not visible. Suboptimal access has major implications for poor outcome, such as a higher risk of damage to healthy adjacent structures, or abandoning the procedure.

Several clinical studies have highlighted the importance of careful patient selection [7, 8]. In a recent study to optimize laryngeal and hypopharyngeal exposure, De Virgilio et al. reported a 100 % success rate in their ability to perform TORS when an examination under anesthetic (EUA) was carried out beforehand. Despite this meticulous approach, failed TORS due to inadequate target exposure has between reported to occur in 7–26 % of cases [9, 10]. Therefore, predictive metrics are a useful adjunct in the preoperative clinical setting to confirm adequate access to the target region and reduce the percentage of unanticipated TORS failures.

Table 7.2 Physical exam findings that should be documented in the preoperative assessment of candidacy for surgery for obstructive sleep apnea hypopnea syndrome [5]

Important physical exam findings
Nasal obstruction
Inter-incisal distance and dentition
Angle class
Friedman palate position
Tonsil size
Modified Cormack–Lehane view
Lingual tonsil size

In a recent cadaver study, three TORS surgeons independently evaluated feasibility using 51 Caucasian cadavers [11]. In order to improve tissue pliability, a phenol–glycerol technique was used to embalm the cadavers. Trans-oral visualization was performed with two retractors commonly used in TORS. Seven anthropometric parameters and the degree of mouth opening were recorded. The results suggest that biometric measures of the extent of mouth-opening, neck circumference, hyoid-mental length, and mandibular body height may provide an important tool in the decision-making process when assessing patient suitability for TORS. The type of retractor used in this study appeared to play an important role in the variability of target exposure. Clinical validation in a large patient cohort is necessary because this study does not account for important factors that affect decision-making in clinical practice such as DISE findings, patient factors (e.g., age and performance status) and surgical experience. When making a clinical decision to proceed with TORS, all of these factors need to be collectively considered to determine patient suitability.

Preoperative cephalometric measurements obtained from preoperative imaging are also useful [12]. Inter-incisor distance and dentition should be carefully assessed. Most patients have an inter-incisal distance greater than 4 cm; less than 2.5 cm generally precludes successful TORS.

For those patients affected by malignant neoplasms, TORS feasibility is qualitatively assessed by performing an examination under anesthesia (EUA) using a mouth gag (Davis-Mayer® Karl Storz, Germany or Boyle-Davis® Surgical Holdings, Essex, UK) or a FK-WO® retractor (Olympus), with the patient in a standardized position (supine with neck extended and head flexed). The EUA includes visualization of the tonsils, tongue base, and supraglottis. Patients with trismus or retrognathia (Angle class II) make the placement of the robotic arms and camera extremely challenging. In patients affected by OSA, if there is marginal accessibility as determined by clinical and cephalometric evaluation, it is suggested that the mouth gag position will be evaluated at the time of DISE to confirm candidacy for TORS.

7.5.3 Friedman Staging System

In an effort to predict success in patients undergoing sleep surgery, Friedman developed a staging system based on tongue position and tonsil size in 2002 [13]; this system has become the standard by which sleep surgeons counsel their patients. The Friedman Staging system categorizes patients based on visualization of the tonsillar pillars, uvula, soft, and hard palate with the oropharynx in a natural position [14]. Tongue position (Grade 1–4) is based on a modification of the Mallampati grade used by anesthesiologists in assessing tongue position; the modification classifies tongue position in the resting position (not protruded) with the mouth wide open. Tonsil size is graded 1–4. Along with BMI, this staging system was developed with the goal of predicting surgical success in patients with OSAHS. In a recent study of patients who undergo TORS ± multilevel procedures for OSAHS, after stratifying by preoperative Friedman stage, success was seen in 75 % of stage I, 70 % of stage

II, 66 % of stage III, and 10 % of stage IV patients. When stratifying by preoperative BMI, success was seen in 75 % of stage II and 72 % of stage III patients with preoperative BMI < 30, compared to 58 % of stage II and 56 % of stage III patients with preoperative BMI > 30 [15].

7.5.4 Modified Cormack–Lehane View

Modified Cormack–Lehane view can also help assess patient candidacy for TORS. The Cormack–Lehane classification was developed as a tool for anesthesiologists as they described the view of the larynx during direct laryngoscopy. A modification has been created using a flexible nasopharygoscope which gives the observer a physiologic view of the anatomy during the awake state [5].

7.5.5 Lingual Tonsil Examination

Grading the size of the lingual tonsil is important in assessing candidacy for surgery. To grade lingual tonsils, the tongue should be in the resting position, with the mouth closed as occurs in sleep. The patient should be in the supine position. Comparison of awake and sedated lingual tonsil size can be done during DISE; however the final grade should be assessed with the patient awake and seated. Lingual tonsils are given a grade of 0–4 (Grade 0 lingual tonsils are not visible or absent, Grade 1 scattered, Grade 2 covers BOT but minimal verticle height, Grade 3 fills vallecula but does not displace epiglottis, Grade 4 fills vallecula and extends above tip of the epiglottis). Grade 3 or 4 upright or supine are considered good surgical candidates. The best candidates for TORS have discrete areas of lingual tonsil hypertrophy low in the vallecula, and/or secondary collapse of the epiglottis due to direct contact with enlarged lingual tonsil. Patients with a large, muscular tongue (Friedman stage 3 or 4) and minimal lingual tonsil tissue are typically poor candidates for TORS. Many of the latter patients also have a BMI > 30; a large tongue is often due to fatty infiltration in obese patients [16].

7.5.6 Body Mass Index

Despite ideal anatomic criteria for TORS, cure of OSAHS in obese patients remains elusive, and surgeons should not raise unrealistic expectations for success in these patients. Vicini et al. were the first authors to show that TORS can show an efficacy of 75 % at 6 months in patients with a body mass index (BMI) under 30, but as BMI increased, the success of TORS fell to 55 % [17]. In a multivariate analysis of over 120 patients who underwent TORS for OSAHS, BMI was shown to predict success (defined as postoperative AHI < 20 and decrease in AHI by 50 %). Patients with a BMI under 30 can expect the best results (86 % of patients show improvement, 69 % have success, 15 % are cured). In fact, operative success was inversely correlated with preoperative BMI as shown in Table 7.3 [3].

It is advisable to encourage obese patients to enter a medical weight loss program while using CPAP prior to surgery. Bariatric surgery may also be an option for these patients. Bariatric surgery is a very effective tool for the treatment of OSAHS, with a success rate of 70 % in a meta-analysis of 12 studies of patients with moderate to severe OSAHS [18]. PSG should be repeated after targeted weight loss has been achieved.

7.6 Drug Induced Sedation Endoscopy

Drug induced sedation endoscopy (DISE) is described in detail in Chap. 6. In brief, it was first described in 1991 by Croft and Pringle and allows the treating physician to observe areas of physical obstruction that occur during induced sleep [19]. The examiner evaluates the airway in a very methodical fashion with the patient both awake and sedated [20]. In 2014, The European Sleep Society presented a position paper and had consensus on many fundamental aspects of DISE, but were unable to agree upon either a unified classification system or a scoring system for DISE. There are two widely used grading systems (VOTE and NOHL). The sites examined include the nasopharynx (velum), oropharynx, hypopharynx (tongue), and larynx or epiglottis (both supraglottic and glottic). For each site, the degree (grade) of obstruction (<25 % grade I, 25–50 % grade II, 50–75 % grade III, and >75 % grade IV), pattern (c = concentric, ap = anterior posterior, l = lateral), and mechanics (vibration, collapse) are recorded. With a better understanding of the multilevel obstruction that characterizes obstructive episodes, surgeons can identify areas that may be amenable to surgical treatment. DISE often reveals areas of obstruction that were not anticipated during office examination and may significantly change the surgical plan [21]. In addition, the patients appreciate the opportunity to review the findings during a separate office consultation, where review of the video and surgical plan is outlined.

Table 7.3 Success in surgery for obstructive sleep apnea hypopnea syndrome (OSAHS) is achieved if the patient obtains a postoperative apnea hypopnea index (AHI) <20 and a decrease from preoperative AHI by 50 %. In a study of 121 patients who underwent transoral robotic surgery for OSAHS, success was inversely correlated with preoperative body mass index. (BMI) [3]

BMI	Success (%)
>30	38.9 (*n* = 36)
<30	56.5 (*n* = 85)
<25	78.3 (*n* = 23)

Table 7.4 Ideal preoperative criteria for patients who wish to undergo transoral robotic surgery (TORS) for obstructive sleep apnea hypopnea syndrome (OSAHS)

Ideal preoperative criteria for TORS
PSG showing moderate to severe OSAHS (AHI > 15)
Age >18 years
BMI < 30
Failed trial of CPAP
Failed surgery
Intraoral accessibility
Identifiable target areas seen on DISE

PSG = polysomnography, BMI = body mass index

7.7 Conclusion

The challenge that has always faced sleep surgeons has been the ability to identify those patients with OSAHS who will benefit from surgery and those who should be counseled to look at other options. Based on the authors' experience as well as a review of the literature, the ideal preoperative criteria for TORS for OSAHS are listed in Table 7.4.

7.8 References

1. Adesanya AO, et al. Perioperative management of obstructive sleep apnea. Chest. 2010;138(6):1489–98.
2. Raveendran R, Chung F. Perioperative consideration of obstructive sleep apnea in ambulatory surgery. Anesthesiol Clin. 2014;32(2):321–8.
3. Hoff PT, Glazer TA, Spector ME. Body mass index predicts success in patients undergoing transoral robotic surgery for obstructive sleep apnea. ORL J Otorhinolaryngol Relat Spec. 2014;76(5):266–72.
4. Siyam MA, Benhamou D. Difficult endotracheal intubation in patients with sleep apnea syndrome. Anesth Analg. 2002;95(4):1098–102. table of contents.
5. Hoff PT, Spector ME. In: Sood M, Leichtle SW, editors. Essentials of robotic surgery. Ann Arbor, MI: Spry Publishing; 2013.
6. Pang KP, Woodson BT. Expansion sphincter pharyngoplasty: a new technique for the treatment of obstructive sleep apnea. Otolaryngol Head Neck Surg. 2007;137(1):110–4.
7. De Virgilio A, Park YM, Kim WS, Baek SJ, Kim SH. How to optimize laryngeal and hypopharyngeal exposure in transoral robotic surgery. Auris Nasus Larynx. 2013;40:312–9.
8. Dowthwaite S, Nichols AC, Yoo J, et al. Transoral robotic total laryngectomy: report of 3 cases. Head Neck. 2013;35(11):E338–42.
9. Vergez S, Lallemant B, Ceruse P, et al. Initial multi-institutional experience with transoral robotic surgery. Otolaryngol Head Neck Surg. 2012;147:475–81.
10. Weinstein GS, O'Malley Jr BW, Magnuson JS, et al. Transoral robotic surgery: a multicenter study to assess feasibility, safety, and surgical margins. Laryngoscope. 2012;122:1701–7.

11. Arora A, Kotecha J, Acharya A, Garas G, Darzi A, Davies DC, Tolley N. Determination of biometric measures to evaluate patient suitability for transoral robotic surgery. Head Neck. 2015;37(9):1254–60.
12. Luginbuhl A, Baker A, Curry J, Drejet S, Miller M, Cognetti D. Preoperative cephalometric analysis to predict transoral robotic surgery exposure. J Robot Surg. 2014;8:313–7.
13. Friedman M, Ibrahim H, Bass L. Clinical staging for sleep-disordered breathing. Otolaryngol Head Neck Surg. 2002;127(1):13–21.
14. Friedman M, et al. Clinical predictors of obstructive sleep apnea. Laryngoscope. 1999;109(12):1901–7.
15. Spector ME, Glazer TA, Hoff PT. Addressing the retrolingual space in moderate to severe obstructive sleep apnea: outcomes stratified by Friedman stage in patients undergoing TORS±multilevel surgery. ORL J Otorhinolaryngol Relat Spec. 2016;78(1):1–8.
16. Nashi N, et al. Lingual fat at autopsy. Laryngoscope. 2007;117(8):1467–73.
17. Vicini C, et al. Transoral robotic surgery of the tongue base in obstructive sleep Apnea–Hypopnea syndrome: anatomic considerations and clinical experience. Head Neck. 2012;34(1):15–22.
18. Greenburg DL, Lettieri CJ, Eliasson AH. Effects of surgical weight loss on measures of obstructive sleep apnea: a meta-analysis. Am J Med. 2009;122(6):535–42.
19. Croft CB, Pringle M. Sleep nasendoscopy: a technique of assessment in snoring and obstructive sleep apnoea. Clin Otolaryngol Allied Sci. 1991;16(5):504–9.
20. Vicini C, et al. The nose oropharynx hypopharynx and larynx (NOHL) classification: a new system of diagnostic standardized examination for OSAHS patients. Eur Arch Otorhinolaryngol. 2012;269(4):1297–300.
21. Campanini A, et al. Awake versus sleep endoscopy: personal experience in 250 OSAHS patients. Acta Otorhinolaryngol Ital. 2010;30(2):73–7.

Part II
Surgery

Chapter 8
Transoral Robotic Surgery as Single Level Surgery for Treatment of Obstructive Sleep Apnea

Ho-Sheng Lin

8.1 Introduction

Since the introduction of uvulopalatopharyngoplasty (UPPP) in the US by Fujita et al. [1], surgical treatment for patients with obstructive sleep apnea/hypopnea syndrome (OSAHS) was mainly directed at the level of the soft palate which was thought to be the main area of obstruction. However, the effectiveness of this surgical procedure was brought into question in a large meta-analysis that showed UPPP to be effective in less than 50 % of the cases [2]. At the same time, surgeons began to realize that OSAHS is a disease entity that is much more complex than previously appreciated. The obstruction may involve multiple levels of the upper airway from the level of nose down to glottis.

Base of tongue (BOT) resection for treatment of OSAHS is not a new concept. Recognizing the important contribution of BOT obstruction in OSAHS, Fujita first reported on the use of carbon dioxide laser for midline glossectomy in 12 patients [3]. Perhaps due to the complexity of the surgery and the potential for major complications, this procedure never became popular.

The increased recognition of BOT as an important site of upper airway obstruction was in part due to the increasing use of sleep endoscopy [4, 5] as a diagnostic tool. As a result of this increased awareness, multiple surgical approaches directed at the BOT level have been described. These techniques included mandibulotomy with genioglossus advancement [6], hyoid advancement [7], Repose® tongue suspension [8], radiofrequency base of tongue reduction (RFBOT) [9], submucosal minimally invasive lingual excision (SMILE) [10], coblation-assisted lingual

H.-S. Lin, M.D. (✉)
Department of Otolaryngology—Head & Neck Surgery, Wayne State University, 4201 St. Antoine St., 5E University Health Center, Detroit, MI 48201, USA

Department of Surgery, John D Dingell VA Medical Center, Detroit, MI, USA
e-mail: hlin@med.wayne.edu

© Springer International Publishing Switzerland 2016

C. Vicini et al. (eds.), *TransOral Robotic Surgery for Obstructive Sleep Apnea*,
DOI 10.1007/978-3-319-34040-1_8

tonsillectomy [11, 12], midline laser glossectomy [3], maxillomandibular advancement (MMA) [13], and implanted upper airway stimulation device [14]. Reports of surgical effectiveness of these procedures vary widely in the literature and are difficult to interpret due to the wide variety of diagnostic and surgical procedures employed, the complexity and uniqueness of the upper airway in individual patients, as well as the varying experience of the reporting surgeons [2, 15].

Transoral robotic surgery (TORS) for resection of oropharyngeal and supraglottic neoplasm was pioneered by Weinstein and O'Malley [16–19] and gained approval by the Food and Drug Administration in December of 2009 for use in the treatment of benign and malignant conditions of oropharynx and larynx. As safety and tolerability of this procedure were established in cancer patients [16, 19], several investigators started to look at the use of this new technology to overcome the limitation of poor visualization and access to the BOT region for treatment of OSAHS [20, 21]. Vicini et al. [20, 22] was the first group to report its experience with TORS-assisted BOT reduction for treatment of OSAHS patients. In a group of 20 patients who underwent variety of upper airway procedures in addition to the TORS-assisted BOT reduction, the mean apnea-hypopnea index (AHI) reduced from 36.3 ± 21.1 to 16.4 ± 15.2 ($p = 0.0001$) [20]. A similar degree of mean AHI reduction [21] was later reported by Friedman et al. in a group of 27 patients who underwent robotically assisted midline glossectomy in conjunction with Z-palatoplasty (ZPP). Despite encouraging results, these reports described the use of TORS-assisted BOT resection in conjunction with other concomitant upper airway procedures making interpretation of the efficacy and contribution of TORS-assisted BOT procedure itself difficult.

We have previously described our experience with 12 patients who underwent TORS-assisted BOT resection without any other concomitant surgical alterations at other levels of upper airway in order to assess the true efficacy of this new procedure alone [23]. We showed significant reduction in AHI, Epworth Sleepiness Scale (ESS), and snoring intensity following TORS-assisted BOT resection alone. Since then, we have continued to offer single level BOT resection in properly selected patients with continued encouraging results.

8.2 Patient Selection via Drug Induced Sleep Endoscopy

Drug induced sleep endoscopy (DISE) as a diagnostic tool has been described in detail elsewhere in this book. Suffice it to say that we have relied heavily on this technique in our practice to localize the site, identify the pattern, and determine the severity of upper airway obstruction.

In review of our data, we found that approximately 30 % of our patients underwent treatment directed only at the BOT level for various reasons. Given the tertiary nature of our practice, we do encounter a sizable number of patients who have previously undergone and failed surgical treatment, most commonly UPPP. Provided that the previously performed UPPP was adequate and provided that the DISE showed the site of obstruction mainly at the BOT level, these patients were offered TORS-assisted BOT procedure alone. Further, in patients who required extensive lateral

BOT resection to involve the inferior tonsillar fossa, we were sufficiently worried about the possibility of circumferential oropharyngeal scarring/stenosis if the BOT resection was performed at the same time as the UPPP. Thus, some of these patients were offered a two-stage approach in which the first stage comprising TORS-assisted BOT resection to be followed, if necessary, by a second stage consisting of other upper airway surgeries such as UPPP. To our surprise, most of these patients never required the second stage procedure because, following the initial BOT surgery, their postoperative PSG showed reduction of AHI to less than 10 with improvement of their daytime symptoms.

Proper patient selection is perhaps one of the most important factors to take into account when considering the applicability of a novel surgical approach. Given the limited data on a small sample size, identification of patient characteristics suitable for this TORS-assisted BOT reduction may not be possible. Despite that, we have previously shown that patient characteristics such as BMI < 30, AHI < 60, and absence of lateral pharyngeal collapse on DISE were associated with improved surgical outcome [24].

8.3 Surgical Technique

The technique for TORS of the BOT has been previously described [16, 19] and is also described in detail elsewhere in this book. Here, we will briefly describe our slightly modified version tailored for OSAHS. Prior to surgery, all patients undergo DISE to evaluate the site of obstruction. The amount and pattern of BOT collapse are carefully analyzed to determine subjectively the extent of tissue resection necessary for each individual patient. The final amount of tissue resected is measured right after the resection by immersing the tissue in saline and measuring the amount saline displaced inside a 120 ml sterile specimen cup. All patients receive perioperative antibiotics and steroid.

In order to avoid distortion of anatomy at the BOT, nasotracheal intubation is routinely performed. To minimize risk of inadvertent airway fire, a wire-reinforced endotracheal tube is used and fraction of inspired oxygen (FiO_2) is kept at less than 30 % if possible. A Leivers® mouth gag (Bausch & Lomb Surgical, Rochester, NY) with Davis-Meyer® tongue blade (Storz, El Segundo, CA) is positioned within the oral cavity to expose the base of tongue. It is important to make sure that the foramen cecum is positioned in the midline of the exposed surgical field to help with orientation. Forward retraction of the tongue is performed with placement of a 2-0 silk over the anterior dorsum of the tongue. It is important to place a tooth guard or some other barrier over the lower dentition in order to avoid laceration of the ventral portion of the tongue.

After fixation of the mouth gag, the robot is rolled in and docked to the right side of the patient at 30° angle to the operating room (OR) table. A 5 mm monopolar spatula, an 8 mm fenestrated bipolar forceps, and an 8.5 mm 0° scope (Intuitive Surgical, Sunnyvale, CA) are then introduced. Placement of the three robotic arms and instruments is carefully optimized to avoid collision and interference during the surgery. Resection then begins in the midline starting from foramen cecum down toward the vallecula posteriorly. The lateral extent of resection is based on the DISE findings and may need to be carried laterally to the inferior tonsillar fossa. Slow and careful dissection using both blunt and sharp dissection is carried out over the lateral base of tongue to avoid injury to the dorsal branch of the lingual artery. If the artery is identified, it is carefully ligated multiple times with clips before dividing. In order to gain improved visualization of BOT tissue posteriorly, the Leivers® mouth gag and 0° scope are replaced with Feyh-Kastenbauer-Weinstein-O'Malley (FK-WO®) retractor (Gyrus Medical, Germany) and 30° scope. Further resection of BOT down to the vallecula and lingual surface of the epiglottis is then carried out.

8.4 Postoperative Care

After removal of the FK-WO® retractor, patients are then taken to the intensive care unit (ICU) intubated. High dose steroid is continued overnight. In the morning following the surgery, patient is allowed to wake up fully and pass the cuff leak test before extubation. Our practice of keeping the patient intubated overnight in the ICU appears to be a compromise between routine tracheostomy by Vicini et al. [20] and extubation at the end of the procedure by Friedman [21]. Patients are kept in the hospital until they can take adequate fluid.

8.5 Surgical Outcomes

We have previously described our experience with 12 patients who underwent TORS-assisted BOT resection without any other concomitant surgical alterations at other levels of upper airway in order to assess the true efficacy of this new procedure alone [23]. We showed significant reduction in AHI (43.9 ± 41.1 to 17.6 ± 16.2, $p = 0.007$), ESS, and snoring intensity following TORS-assisted BOT resection alone. Six of 12 patients (50 %) achieved surgical success response and all have postoperative AHI of less than 10 (range 0.5–9.3). Since then, we have continued to offer single level BOT resection in properly selected patients. Analysis of this larger sample ($n = 22$) showed that the AHI reduction continued to be significant (45.9 ± 34.3 preoperatively to 21.3 ± 19.9 postoperatively, $p = 0.001$, unpublished data) with 11 out of 22 patients (50 %) achieving surgical success with AHI < 15 and ESS < 10.

8.6 Complications

Complications associated with TORS-assisted BOT reduction are also described elsewhere in this book. The main issues that we have encountered in our practice included taste disturbance, oropharyngeal stenosis, and bleeding.

Taste disturbance is a well-known complication following any oral procedure. In one large study involving 223 post-tonsillectomy patients, 15 (8 %) patients complain of subjective taste disturbance 6 months following tonsillectomy. On longer term follow-up, 2 (0.9 %) patients reported persistent dysgeusia at 21 months and 54 months following tonsillectomy [25]. Although the etiology for this complication following TORS-assisted BOT resection for OSAHS is largely unknown, possible causes include direct surgical injury to the taste buds in the BOT as well as compression and stretching injury to the branches of lingual nerve from the prolonged retraction during surgery. It is therefore important that the surgeon periodically relaxes the retractor during the case and that the patients be informed of this possible complication prior to the surgery. Fortunately, in our experience, the taste disturbance typically resolves within a few months in the majority of our patients.

Another complication that we encountered early in our experience is oropharyngeal stenosis due to scarring of BOT to tonsillar bed. These patients complained of dysphagia with solid food and typically required another surgery to release the scar tissue. Periodic Kenalog® injection in the office may also help in prevention of recurrence of stenosis. In order to avoid this complication, we would recommend that a two-stage approach be considered for patients who required extensive lateral BOT resection to involve the inferior tonsillar fossa.

Due to the absence of a reliable and constant anatomic landmark, surgical intervention in the BOT can be burdened with the potential devastating complication of injuring the critical hypoglossal/lingual artery neurovascular bundle (HLNVB). Thus, familiarity with anatomy of the HLNVB is critically important. The average distance from the foramen cecum to the HLNVB was found to be 1.66 ± 0.25 cm in a cadaver study [26] and 1.68 ± 0.21 cm in a study using computed tomographic angiography [27]. Thus, functional surgery performed within approximately 1.5 cm of the foramen cecum should be safe. Meticulous dissection should be carried out over the lateral tongue to avoid injury to the dorsal branch of the lingual artery.

8.7 Concluding Remarks

Although we demonstrate the effectiveness of TORS-assisted BOT resection as a stand-alone surgical modality in the treatment of OSAHS in some of our patients, we do not necessarily advocate the use of this surgical technique alone for treatment of OSAHS. No single surgical procedure is perfect and it is incumbent upon the surgeon to identify and select the most optimal procedure or combination of procedures to treat the anatomic obstruction unique to each OSAHS patients. A recently published meta-analysis [28] found that there is currently insufficient data to evaluate the role of glossectomy as a standalone procedure for the treatment of OSAHS. Thus, although the preliminary result on the use of TORS-assisted BOT resection for the treatment of patients with OSAHS is encouraging, its use as a stand-alone procedure cannot be advocated at this time. Further investigations are warranted and more studies need to be performed to further evaluate the efficacy, benefits, and limitations of this new technique.

References

1. Fujita S, Conway W, Zorick F, Roth T. Surgical correction of anatomic abnormalities in obstructive sleep apnea syndrome: uvulopalatopharyngoplasty. Otolaryngol Head Neck Surg. 1981;89:923–34.
2. Sher AE, Schechtman KB, Piccirillo JF. The efficacy of surgical modifications of the upper airway in adults with obstructive sleep apnea syndrome. Sleep. 1996;19:156–77.
3. Fujita S, Woodson BT, Clark JL, Wittig R. Laser midline glossectomy as a treatment for obstructive sleep apnea. Laryngoscope. 1991;101:805–9.
4. Soares D, Sinawe H, Folbe AJ, et al. Lateral oropharyngeal wall and supraglottic airway collapse associated with failure in sleep apnea surgery. Laryngoscope. 2012;122:473–9.
5. Ravesloot MJ, de Vries N. One hundred consecutive patients undergoing drug-induced sleep endoscopy: results and evaluation. Laryngoscope. 2011;121:2710–6.
6. Riley RW, Powell NB, Guilleminault C. Maxillofacial surgery and obstructive sleep apnea: a review of 80 patients. Otolaryngol Head Neck Surg. 1989;101:353–61.
7. Riley RW, Powell NB, Guilleminault C. Obstructive sleep apnea and the hyoid: a revised surgical procedure. Otolaryngol Head Neck Surg. 1994;111:717–21.
8. Woodson BT. A tongue suspension suture for obstructive sleep apnea and snorers. Otolaryngol Head Neck Surg. 2001;124:297–303.
9. Woodson BT, Nelson L, Mickelson S, Huntley T, Sher A. A multi-institutional study of radiofrequency volumetric tissue reduction for OSAS. Otolaryngol Head Neck Surg. 2001;125:303–11.
10. Maturo SC, Mair EA. Submucosal minimally invasive lingual excision: an effective, novel surgery for pediatric tongue base reduction. Ann Otol Rhinol Laryngol. 2006;115:624–30.
11. Lin AC, Koltai PJ. Persistent pediatric obstructive sleep apnea and lingual tonsillectomy. Otolaryngol Head Neck Surg. 2009;141:81–5.
12. Rotenberg B, Tan S. Endoscopic-assisted radiofrequency lingual tonsillectomy. Laryngoscope. 2011;121:994–6.
13. Riley RW, Powell NB, Guilleminault C. Obstructive sleep apnea syndrome: a review of 306 consecutively treated surgical patients. Otolaryngol Head Neck Surg. 1993;108:117–25.
14. Van de Heyning PH, Badr MS, Baskin JZ, et al. Implanted upper airway stimulation device for obstructive sleep apnea. Laryngoscope. 2012;122:1626–33.
15. Caples SM, Rowley JA, Prinsell JR, et al. Surgical modifications of the upper airway for obstructive sleep apnea in adults: a systematic review and meta-analysis. Sleep. 2010;33:1396–407.
16. Weinstein GS, O'Malley BW, Cohen MA, Quon H. Transoral robotic surgery for advanced oropharyngeal carcinoma TORS for advanced oropharyngeal carcinoma. Arch Otolaryngol Head Neck Surg. 2010;136:1079–85.
17. Weinstein GS, O'Malley Jr BW, Snyder W, Hockstein NG. Transoral robotic surgery: supraglottic partial laryngectomy. Ann Otol Rhinol Laryngol. 2007;116:19–23.
18. Weinstein GS, O'Malley Jr BW, Snyder W, Sherman E, Quon H. Transoral robotic surgery: radical tonsillectomy. Arch Otolaryngol Head Neck Surg. 2007;133:1220–6.
19. O'Malley Jr BW, Weinstein GS, Snyder W, Hockstein NG. Transoral robotic surgery (TORS) for base of tongue neoplasms. Laryngoscope. 2006;116:1465–72.
20. Vicini C, Dallan I, Canzi P, et al. Transoral robotic surgery of the tongue base in obstructive sleep apnea-hypopnea syndrome: anatomic considerations and clinical experience. Head Neck. 2012;34:15–22.
21. Friedman M, Hamilton C, Samuelson CG, et al. Transoral robotic glossectomy for the treatment of obstructive sleep apnea-hypopnea syndrome. Otolaryngol Head Neck Surg. 2012;146:854–62.
22. Vicini C, Dallan I, Canzi P, Frassineti S, La Pietra MG, Montevecchi F. Transoral robotic tongue base resection in obstructive sleep apnoea-hypopnoea syndrome: a preliminary report. ORL J Otorhinolaryngol Relat Spec. 2010;72:22–7.

23. Lin HS, Rowley JA, Badr MS, et al. Transoral robotic surgery for treatment of obstructive sleep apnea-hypopnea syndrome. Laryngoscope. 2013;123:1811–6.
24. Lin HS, Rowley JA, Folbe AJ, Yoo GH, Badr MS, Chen W. Transoral robotic surgery for treatment of obstructive sleep apnea: factors predicting surgical response. Laryngoscope. 2015;125:1013–20.
25. Heiser C, Landis BN, Giger R, et al. Taste disorders after tonsillectomy: a long-term follow-up. Laryngoscope. 2012;122:1265–6.
26. Lauretano AM, Li KK, Caradonna DS, Khosta RK, Fried MP. Anatomic location of the tongue base neurovascular bundle. Laryngoscope. 1997;107:1057–9.
27. Hou T, Shao J, Fang S. The definition of the V zone for the safety space of functional surgery of the tongue. Laryngoscope. 2012;122:66–70.
28. Murphey AW, Kandl JA, Nguyen SA, Weber AC, Gillespie MB. The effect of glossectomy for obstructive sleep apnea: a systematic review and meta-analysis. Otolaryngol Head Neck Surg. 2015;153:334–42.

Chapter 9
TORS in a Multilevel Procedure

Ahmed Bahgat, Ehsan Hendawy, Kenny P. Pang, and Claudio Vicini

9.1 Introduction

Historically, multilevel procedures for the surgical therapy of obstructive sleep apnea (OSA) were presented for the first time in 1989 by Waite et al. [1]. The authors combined nasal surgery with a uvulopalatopharyngoplasty (UPPP), transoral tongue surgery, genioglossus advancement (GA), and maxillo-mandibular advancement osteotomy (MMA).

Fujita et al. [2] presented classification of the upper airway into different levels of obstruction, either retropalatal, retrolingual, or combined retropalatal and retrolingual obstruction. On the basis of this distinction, Riley et al. [3] defined the term and concept of multilevel surgery.

Current surgical management of obstructive sleep apnea (OSA) is most successfully achieved by multilevel surgery [4]. This was confirmed after thorough understanding of the complexity of airway obstruction by drug-induced sleep endoscopy (DISE) that showed that the hypopharynx and base of tongue, not only the palate, are important anatomic components of obstruction in OSA [5]. In addition, the lateral collapse of the airway has been noted to be of particular significance in recalcitrant cases [4].

A. Bahgat, M.D., M.Sc., E.B.E. (✉)
Department of Otorhinolaryngology—Head & Neck Surgery, Alexandria University, Alexandria, Egypt
e-mail: ahmedyassinbahgat@gmail.com

E. Hendawy, M.B., B.Ch.
Department of Otolaryngology, Head-Neck Surgery, University of Zagazig, Zagazig, Egypt

K.P. Pang, M.B.B.S., M.R.C.S., F.R.C.S.
Department of Otolaryngology, Asia Sleep Centre, Paragon Medical, Singapore, Singapore
e-mail: drkpang@gmail.com

C. Vicini, M.D.
Head and Neck Department - ENT & Oral Surgery Unit - G.B. Morgagni - L. Pierantoni Hospital, Forlì – Infermi Hospital, Faenza - ASL of Romagna, Italy

© Springer International Publishing Switzerland 2016

C. Vicini et al. (eds.), *TransOral Robotic Surgery for Obstructive Sleep Apnea*,
DOI 10.1007/978-3-319-34040-1_9

9.2 Historical Background

Vicini et al. [6, 7] reported on their experience with 20 patients who underwent TORS-assisted tongue base reduction concomitantly with multiple other procedures such as septoplasty, supraglottoplasty, UPPP, turbinate reduction, and ethmoidectomy. In this group, the mean AHI dropped from 36.3±21.1 to 16.4±15.2 ($P = 0.0001$), and mean ESS dropped from 12.6±4.4 to 7.7±3.3 postoperatively ($P = 0.0003$) [6]. The failures regarding the AHI, in this group, were assumed to be related to the fact that the oropharyngeal region was not treated properly. More specifically, in certain patients, TORS failed because the epiglottis and the oropharynx were not addressed surgically; after TORS, these two regions continued to demonstrate collapse [7].

Friedman reported on 27 patients who underwent robotic-assisted midline glossectomy in conjunction with Z-palatoplasty (ZPP). The mean AHI dropped from 54.6±21.8 to 18.6±9.1 ($P < 0.001$) and mean ESS dropped from 14.4±4.5 to 5.4±3.1 postoperatively ($P < 0.001$) [8].

Lin et al. reported the clinical and polysomnographic outcome of 12 patients who underwent TORS-assisted BOT resection alone without any other concomitant surgical interventions. It was the first study looking at the efficacy of TORS to address obstruction at the level of BOT only, not confounded by surgical alterations at other levels of the airway. A significant reduction in AHI, ESS, and snoring intensity following TORS-assisted BOT resection was noted [9].

Between 2008 and 2014 more than 100 cases have been published from seven different centers around the world. In 2014 the first multicenter study about TORS in which a cohort of 243 cases from seven groups in five different countries was available [10].

In 2015, Thaler et al. [4] conducted a study using DISE to show the importance of adding TORS in a multilevel procedure on degree of reduction of AHI. Seventy-five patients completed DISE, TORS for OSA, UPPP, and pre- and postoperative polysomnography. The mean age of patients was 49.7 years; the mean preoperative BMI was 32.3. Patients were further divided into two groups for purposes of comparison: those who had had no prior pharyngeal surgery and those who had had prior pharyngeal surgery (this included tonsillectomy and UPPP). The best outcomes were obtained in those patients who had had no prior surgery and who underwent TORS in addition to UPPP (67 % reduction in AHI versus 33 % for UPPP alone) [4].

9.3 Effect of Palate Surgery on TORS Results

Vicini et al. have performed 160 cases of TORS for OSA between May 2008 and April 2014. In the beginning, all the palate surgeries were treated performing a classic UPPP. Since June 2010, the UPPP palate technique has in most cases been replaced by a modified expansion sphincter pharyngoplasty, inspired by the Pang expansion sphincter pharyngoplasty technique [11]. For that reason, our group has had the unique opportunity to compare the contribution of two different palate surgeries (UPPP and ESP) to the outcome of a multilevel, one-step procedure including a TORS tongue base reduction (TBR) and supraglottoplasty (SGP) [12].

9.3.1 *Expansion Sphincter Pharyngoplasty*

Two groups of 12 severe OSAHS cases each were sorted according to the primary selection criteria of statistically comparable preoperative AHI (AHI = 38 in both groups). The two groups were also reasonably matched for sex, age, body mass index (BMI), and volume of removed tongue base (TB) tissue. Both groups underwent multilevel surgery of the upper airway including nose surgery if required and TORS TBR-SGP according to the Vicini–Montevecchi technique [6]. Meanwhile, patients in Group A underwent UPPP procedure according to the Fairbanks technique [13], while patients in Group B underwent expansion sphincter pharyngoplasty (ESP) using a modification of the Pang–Woodson technique [11]. These modifications include (1) blunt palate tunneling without mucosal incisions; (2) posterior pillar flap tip stay suture in order to prevent a possible tearing of the tip by the pulling suture; and (3) systematic use of a second intermediate suturing of the flap under direct visual control [12].

The purpose of the study was to show the superiority of ESP compared to the traditional UPPP as a multilevel procedure. The most striking finding is a postoperative AHI of 9.9 ± 8.6 SD for the ESP group versus a postoperative AHI of 19.8 ± 14.1 SD for the UPPP group. Pre- and postoperative comparison, in terms of AHI, reached statistical significance for both techniques. Comparison between UPPP and ESP, in terms of AHI improvement, is at the limit of statistical significance [12].

The authors concluded that the palate component of multilevel procedure, ESP, including conventional nose surgery and robotically assisted TB-SPG surgery, seems to be superior to UPPP. Functional and objective superiority (as measured by postoperative polysomnography) and better acceptance by the patient (less pain and less late discomfort) seem to balance the longer surgical time, the higher technical complexity, and the longer learning curve [12].

9.3.2 *Barbed Reposition Pharyngoplasty*

A systematic retrospective review of the literature, analysis of our cases, and a targeted cadaver dissection study prompted us to modify our approach to the lateral pharyngeal wall switching from ESP to relocation pharyngoplasty (RP) according to Li et al. [14] with some modifications [15]. The new technique includes the following: (1) a “barbed” suture, which refers to the use of knotless, bidirectional, and re-absorbable sutures introduced for similar purposes by Mantovani et al. [16]; (2) "reposition pharyngoplasty" which displaces the posterior pillar (palatopharyngeal muscle) in an anterior-lateral position to enlarge the oropharyngeal inlet as well as the retro-palatal space; (3) suspension of the posterior pillar to the pterygo-mandibular raphe; and (4) weakening of the inferior aspect of the palatopharyngeal muscle by means of a partial horizontal transection. The multiple sustaining suture loops of barbed reposition pharyngoplasty (BRP) proved to be more stable than the single pulling tip suture of ESP, with minimal risk of tearing the muscle fibers and losing the suspension force.

In a preliminary study of ten adult male patients undergoing multilevel surgery including BRP (mean age 53.4 ± 12.4, mean BMI 28.5 ± 3.6), the preoperative AHI was reduced from 43.65 ± 26.83 to 13.57 ± 15.41 ($P = 0.007$), and the preoperative ESS was reduced from 11.6 ± 4.8 to 4.3 ± 2 ($P < 0.01$) [15].

The most important advantage of this palatal technique is the stability of the new expanded retro-palatal space, which was confirmed 6 months postoperatively by in-office fiber-optic examination. In addition, this technique is easily taught, and operative time is short, decreasing over the course of the study to as short as 20 min. Finally, pain as assessed by visual analog scale (VAS) and dysphagia as assessed by MD-Anderson dysphagia questionnaire showed that this technique is well tolerated by patients who undergo multilevel surgery including TORS—TBR and SGP [15].

References

1. Waite PD, Wooten V, Lachner J, Guyette RF. Maxillomandibular advancement surgery in 23 patients with obstructive sleep apnea syndrome. J Oral Maxillofac Surg. 1989;47(12):1256–61. discussion 62.
2. Fujita S. Obstructive sleep apnea syndrome: pathophysiology, upper airway evaluation and surgical treatment. Ear Nose Throat J. 1993;72(1):67–72. 5–6.
3. Riley RW, Powell NB, Guilleminault C. Obstructive sleep apnea syndrome: a review of 306 consecutively treated surgical patients. Otolaryngol Head Neck Surg. 1993;108(2):117–25.
4. Thaler ER, Rassekh CH, Lee JM, Weinstein GS, O'Malley Jr BW. Outcomes for multilevel surgery for sleep apnea: obstructive sleep apnea, transoral robotic surgery, and uvulopalatopharyngoplasty. Laryngoscope. 2016;126(1):266–9.
5. Kezirian EJ. Nonresponders to pharyngeal surgery for obstructive sleep apnea: insights from drug-induced sleep endoscopy. Laryngoscope. 2011;121(6):1320–6.
6. Vicini C, Dallan I, Canzi P, Frassineti S, Nacci A, Seccia V, et al. Transoral robotic surgery of the tongue base in obstructive sleep apnea-hypopnea syndrome: anatomic considerations and clinical experience. Head Neck. 2012;34(1):15–22.
7. Vicini C, Dallan I, Canzi P, Frassineti S, La Pietra MG, Montevecchi F. Transoral robotic tongue base resection in obstructive sleep apnoea-hypopnoea syndrome: a preliminary report. ORL J Otorhinolaryngol Relat Spec. 2010;72(1):22–7.
8. Friedman M, Hamilton C, Samuelson CG, Kelley K, Taylor D, Pearson-Chauhan K, et al. Transoral robotic glossectomy for the treatment of obstructive sleep apnea-hypopnea syndrome. Otolaryngol Head Neck Surg. 2012;146(5):854–62.
9. Lin HS, Rowley JA, Badr MS, Folbe AJ, Yoo GH, Victor L, et al. Transoral robotic surgery for treatment of obstructive sleep apnea-hypopnea syndrome. Laryngoscope. 2013;123(7): 1811–6.

10. Vicini C, Montevecchi F, Campanini A, Dallan I, Hoff PT, Spector ME, et al. Clinical outcomes and complications associated with TORS for OSAHS: a benchmark for evaluating an emerging surgical technology in a targeted application for benign disease. ORL J Otorhinolaryngol Relat Spec. 2014;76(2):63–9.
11. Pang KP, Woodson BT. Expansion sphincter pharyngoplasty: a new technique for the treatment of obstructive sleep apnea. Otolaryngol Head Neck Surg. 2007;137(1):110–4.
12. Vicini C, Montevecchi F, Pang K, Bahgat A, Dallan I, Frassineti S, et al. Combined transoral robotic tongue base surgery and palate surgery in obstructive sleep apnea-hypopnea syndrome: expansion sphincter pharyngoplasty versus uvulopalatopharyngoplasty. Head Neck. 2014;36(1):77–83.
13. Fairbanks DN. Operative techniques of uvulopalatopharyngoplasty. Ear Nose Throat J. 1999;78(11):846–50.
14. Li HY, Lee LA. Relocation pharyngoplasty for obstructive sleep apnea. Laryngoscope. 2009;119(12):2472–7.
15. Vicini C, Hendawy E, Campanini A, Eesa M, Bahgat A, AlGhamdi S, Montevecchi F, et al. Barbed reposition pharyngoplasty (BRP) for OSAHS: a feasibility, safety, efficacy and teachability pilot study. "We are on the giant's shoulders". Eur Arch Otorhinolaryngol. 2015;272(10):3065–70.
16. Mantovani M, Minetti A, Torretta S, Pincherle A, Tassone G, Pignataro L. The "Barbed Roman Blinds" technique: a step forward. Acta Otorhinolaryngol Ital. 2013;33(2):128.

Chapter 10
Alternative Procedures

Mohamed Eesa, Ahmed Bahgat, and Ehsan Hendawy

10.1 Introduction

TORS was devised as a robotically assisted transoral version of Chabolle's operation (open transcervical Tongue Base Reduction and Hyo-Epiglottoplasty, TBRHE) [1] for moderate to severe obstructive sleep apnea hypopnea syndrome (OSAHS). This chapter gives an overview of the alternative procedures that can be used to address tongue base obstruction in OSAHS patients.

10.2 Historical Background

The ideal surgical approach for the tongue base should provide both excellent exposure and visualization in order to perform a safe and adequate resection of obstructing tissue. The procedure should minimize collateral damage to surroundings structures in order to maintain the critical role of the tongue base in determining the patient's quality of life.

Base of tongue (BOT) resection for the treatment of OSAHS is not a new concept. In 1991, Fujita et al. first reported on the use of carbon dioxide laser for midline glossectomy in 12 patients who did not respond to UPPP [2]. Many modifications of this technique have been published to improve the response rate; however, surgical management of the tongue base by a microscopic-laser-assisted approach is

M. Eesa, M.D., M.Sc., E.B.E. (✉) • E. Hendawy, M.D., M.Sc., E.B.E.
Department of Otolaryngology and Head-Neck Surgery, University of Zagazig,
Zagazig 44519, Sharkia, Egypt
e-mail: dr.eesaorl@gmail.com; ehsanhendawy@gmail.com

A. Bahgat, M.D., M.Sc., E.B.E.
Department of Otorhinolaryngology—Head & Neck Surgery, Alexandria University,
Alexandria, Egypt

© Springer International Publishing Switzerland 2016

C. Vicini et al. (eds.), *TransOral Robotic Surgery for Obstructive Sleep Apnea*,
DOI 10.1007/978-3-319-34040-1_10

challenging from a technical point and requires extensive training. Furthermore, using this technique, manipulation of tongue base tissues causes complex geometric distortions in the architecture of the region, thus impairing the surgeon's orientation and increasing the risk of complications. Insufficient visualization of crucial neurovascular structures restricts resection to the midline of the tongue, ignoring the lateral tongue base. In addition, the postoperative functional and pain profiles for laser resection are very problematic. These are the reasons why laser resections were abandoned in many parts of the world.

Open approaches through the neck can be performed to improve access, but have significant associated morbidity. Historically, Chabolle was the first to propose a tongue base resection through a transcervical suprahyoid approach. Later, Vicini et al. [3] modified this technique to include a transcervical infra-hyoid submucosal tongue base reduction with the addition of thyro-hyoidopexy to improve its effectiveness and reduce complications. Although the open approach is effective, the procedures remained confined to a very limited number of centers due to both the technical difficulties and associated morbidity.

In recent times, reasonable success has been achieved through the use of radiofrequency base-of-tongue reduction (RFBOT) through either a transoral or transcervical ultrasound-guided approach; however, radiofrequency surgery can only be successful in cases of moderate tongue base hypertrophy [4].

Submucosal minimally invasive lingual excision (SMILE), and Coblation® assisted lingual tonsillectomy with or without endoscopic assistance have been described to address large tongue base obstruction in children with obstructive macroglossia and has been found to be promising. However, these procedures are limited by poor visualization and access to the BOT region. Moreover, SMILE is believed to be more invasive and has resulted in increased morbidity as compared to RFBOT; the most significant potential complication of SMILE is damage to the lingual artery or the hypoglossal nerve.

10.3 TORS Versus Chabolle's Operation

A retrospective comparative study was carried out in our center to compare TORS versus transcervical tongue base reduction (according to Chabolle); two matched groups of OSAHS patients were sorted according to the primary selection criteria of statistically comparable preoperative AHI. The two groups were also reasonably matched for sex, age, body mass index (BMI), and palate surgery (UPPP). Tracheostomy was done in all patients.

Postoperative AHI registered (after at least 6 months) showed no statistically significant difference ($p = 0.14$) between TORS (14.21 ± 10.46) and Chabolle procedure (21.67 ± 19.38). The same result was obtained in ESS; 7.75 ± 3.52 for Chabolle procedure, and 6.91 ± 4.22 for TORS ($p = 0.5$).

In conclusion, TORS can achieve the same effect as the Chabolle operation both subjectively (ESS) and objectively (AHI) with significantly less operative time (182.5 ± 51.72 min for Chabolle and 150.35 ± 36.59 min for TORS), less invasiveness (no cervical incision), less postoperative hospital stay (19.92 ± 8.19 days for

Chabolle and 7.68 ± 1.91 days for TORS), and an earlier resumption of oral feeding (11.83 ± 7.94 days for Chabolle and 1.13 ± 0.34 days for TORS). The total cost between TORS and Chabolle was statistically insignificant (5494.98 € for Chabolle and 5572.78 € for TORS) ($p > 0.05$) due to less operative time and less postoperative hospital stay for TORS patients.

10.4 TORS Versus Maxillomandibular Advancement (MMA)

A retrospective comparative study was carried out in our center to compare TORS versus MMA (unpublished data); two matched groups of OSAHS patients were sorted according to the primary selection criteria of statistically comparable preoperative AHI. The two groups were also reasonably matched for sex, age, and body mass index (BMI); tracheostomy was performed in all patients.

Postoperative AHI registered (after at least 6 months) showed a statistically significant difference ($p = 0.02$) between TORS (14.21 ± 10.46) and MMA (8.16 ± 6.98). However, there was no statistically significant difference in postoperative ESS; 7.68 ± 1.34 for MMA and 6.91 ± 4.22 for TORS ($p = 0.5$).

There was a significant difference in favor of TORS in total operative time (357.6 ± 41.48 min for MMA and 150.35 ± 36.59 min for TORS), start of oral feeding (16 ± 1.32 days for MMA and 1.13 ± 0.34 days for TORS), and total cost (10,702.08 € for MMA including cost of titanium plates and screws used in fixation, and 5572.78 € for TORS).

Moreover, TORS was found to be BMI sensitive; when comparing two matched groups with BMI greater than 30, results of MMA are superior to TORS for postoperative AHI (7.94 ± 6.68 for MMA and 18.74 ± 13.12 for TORS). But when comparing the groups with a BMI equal or less than 30, there is no significant difference in postoperative AHI between TORS and MMA (8.63 ± 8.05 for Bi-max and 12.34 ± 10.29 for TORS).

10.5 TORS Versus Genioglossus Advancement ± Hyoid Suspension

Three groups of patients who underwent tongue base surgery, including TORS, genioglossus advancement (GGA) with or without hyoid suspension (HS), and hyoid suspension alone were evaluated (unpublished data). The three groups were matched for AHI sex, age, BMI, and palate surgery.

Postoperative AHI registered (after at least 6 months) was 28.28 ± 23.72 for GGA ± HS group, 21.04 ± 16.55 for the HS group and 14.13 ± 11.72 for the TORS group. The difference in postoperative AHI was statistically significant between TORS versus either GGA ± HS ($p = 0.008$) or hyoid suspension groups ($p = 0.04$) in favor of TORS. However, the difference was not statistically significant between

GGA±HS and the HS groups ($p=0.18$). In conclusion, the AHI reduction in TORS is better than GGA±HS or HS alone (unpublished data).

Postoperative improvement of ESS showed the same results (9.5±1.74 for GGA±HS group, 7.72±2.33 for HS group and 6.33±3.15 for the TORS group). The difference in postoperative ESS was statistically significant between TORS compared to either GGA±HS ($p=0.001$) or HS groups ($p=0.02$) in favor of TORS. In summary, ESS reduction in TORS is better than HS or GGA±HS.

GGA±HS has proven to be inferior to TORS in terms of both subjective and objective functional outcomes.

Hyoid suspension as performed in our institution as thyro-hyoidopexy (THP) moves the hyoid and, subsequently, the tongue base anteriorly. Its primary function is to stent the lateral hypopharyngeal walls and prevent lateral collapse in moderate OSAHS patients (AHI less than 30). THP should be avoided if the main pattern of hypopharyngeal collapse, as seen by DISE, is anterior–posterior as is often observed in severe OSAHS patients (AHI greater than 30), in which case TORS would be recommended. Performing both THP and TORS as a single procedure may result in the development of a pharyngo-cutaneous fistula and is therefore not advised. If TORS BOT resection is unsuccessful and lateral hypopharyngeal collapse is present on DISE, THP is currently under evaluation as a salvage procedure.

10.6 Hypoglossal Nerve Stimulation

Hypoglossal nerve stimulation (HGNS) returns tone to the sleeping tongue. A number of animal studies, conducted in multiple labs and reported over the past several years, have demonstrated that hypoglossal nerve stimulation can produce consistent improvements in the tone of the tongue [5]. Selective neural stimulation would appear to offer advantages. For example, upper airway resistance can be decreased by stimulating either the geniohyoid muscle [6] or the medial genioglossus [7]. In addition, airway compliance can be increased by stimulation of the hyoglossus and styloglossus muscles. This has been demonstrated in animals and in humans.

Early studies were conducted in patients where unilateral hypoglossal nerve stimulators were implanted in eight patients [8]. No surgical complications were reported. As reported by the authors, all of the patients derived significant clinical benefit over a follow-up period of 6 months. The study demonstrated the feasibility and therapeutic potential for hypoglossal nerve stimulation in obstructive sleep apnea in man. More recent studies of neurostimulation devices for OSA have been completed in larger populations with success.

A single-arm, open-label study has been completed in four sites in Australia using the HGNS device manufactured by Apnex Medical®, Inc. Twenty-one subjects with moderate to severe OSA were enrolled. The results showed significant improvement (all $p<0.05$) from baseline to 6 months in: AHI (43.1±17.5 to 19.5±16.7), ESS (12.1±4.7 to 8.1±4.4). Two serious device-related adverse events occurred. In conclusion, the HGNS demonstrated favorable safety, efficacy, and compliance [9].

Another clinical study was completed by Inspire Medical Systems®, Inc. Patients with moderate to severe OSA were implanted. The study was conducted in two parts.

In Part 1, patients were enrolled with broad selection criteria. In Part 2, patients were enrolled using selection criteria derived from the experience in Part 1. In Part 1, responders had both a BMI≤32 and AHI≤50 ($p<0.05$) with predominate hypopnea-based OSA and did not have complete concentric palatal collapse. Part 2 patients were selected using responder criteria and showed an improvement of AHI from baseline 38.9±9.8 to 10.0±11.0 ($p<0.01$) at 6 months post-implant. Subjective measures improved significantly in Part 1 and 2 subjects. This study has demonstrated that therapy with upper airway stimulation is safe and efficacious in a select group (predominate hypopnea without complete concentric palatal collapse) of patients with moderate to severe OSA who cannot or will not use CPAP as primary treatment [10].

Imthera Medical® completed a prospective, feasibility study at a single center in Belgium to assess the safety and preliminary efficacy of the aura6000™ Targeted Hypoglossal Neurostimulation Sleep Therapy System (aura6000). Thirteen subjects were implanted and completed the 12-month follow-up visit. The mean AHI dropped from 45.2±17.8 at screening to 21.0±16.5 at 12 months (53.5 % mean improvement). Similarly, the mean oxygen desaturation index (ODI) dropped from 29.2±19.6 to 15.3±16.2 at 12 months (47.6 % mean improvement). Three of the patients in the study were nonresponders and they had either a large uvula, BMI>37, or central sleep apnea [11].

Recently, a multicenter study using the Imthera® system has been conducted in nine medical centers over Europe and the USA. The results are not yet published, but in well-selected candidates the treatment showed promising results.

10.6.1 Basic Design

The basic design of HGNS device (Inspire® and Apnex®) required a more distal electrode placement to direct the stimulation to the branch of the hypoglossal nerve that controls the genioglossus muscle, and a respiration sensor to synchronize stimulation with inspiration to mitigate muscle fatigue. By comparison, the Imthera aura6000 System® uses a programmable, multi-current source stimulator and multi-contact electrode. This design permits a more proximal electrode placement on the hypoglossal nerve (HGN) where seven hemi-tongue muscles can be stimulated, and employs targeted stimulation of a subset of the HGN to produce tonus in the posterior tongue. The design cycles stimulation between muscles to preclude muscle fatigue, with no need of a respiratory sensor.

10.6.2 Additional Remarks on Therapy by HGNS

- The initial response to stimulation is almost always a predictor for the long lasting success, which means that if the patient does not achieve a good response the early months of therapy, it is most probable that he or she will not obtain any improvement with continuation of therapy.
- The device is more effective in patient with hypopnea rather than complete obstruction.

- Drug induced sleep endoscopy (DISE) is required to detect the presence of complete circular palatal collapse during DISE which is a negative predictor for therapeutic success (Vanderveken et al. [12]).
- Furthermore, we believe that it is better to apply stimulation therapy to muscular tongue base obstruction. Hypopharyngeal obstruction due to localized lymphoid hyperplasia can be easily addressed by TORS.
- HGNS has the same concept of multilevel one stage surgery because it can resolve multilevel collapse not only in the area of the tongue base but also at the level of the palate.
- Patient selection is crucial due to the high cost of the device. Selection criteria are listed below according to our experience and according to previous studies:
  - BMI < 32.
  - Tonsils size 1–2
  - Friedman palate position less than 3
  - AHI < 50 (predominance of hypopnea rather than apnea)
  - Patients without complete circular collapse at the level of the palate.

References

1. Chabolle F, Wagner I, Blumen MB, et al. Tongue base reduction with hyoepigottoplasty: a treatment for severe obstructive sleep apnea. Laryngoscope. 1999;109(8):1273–80.
2. Fujita S, Woodson BT, Clark JL, Wittig R. Laser midline glossectomy as a treatment for obstructive sleep apnea. Laryngoscope. 1991;101(8):805–9.
3. Vicini C, Frassineti S, La Pietra MG, De Vito A, Dallan I, Canzi P. Tongue base reduction with thyro-hyoido-pexy (TBRTHP) vs. tongue base reduction with hyo-epiglottoplasty (TBRHE) in mild-severe OSAHS adult treatment. Preliminary findings from a prospective randomised trial. Acta Otorhinolaryngol Ital. 2010;30(3):144–8.
4. Blumen MB, Coquille F, Rocchicioli C, Mellot F, Chabolle F. Radiofrequency tongue reduction through a cervical approach: a pilot study. Laryngoscope. 2006;116(10):1887–93.
5. Fuller DD, Williams JS, Janssen PL, Fregosi RF. Effect of co-activation of tongue protrudor and retractor muscles on tongue movements and pharyngeal airflow mechanics in the rat. J Physiol. 1999;519(Pt.2):601–13.
6. Oliven A, Schnall RP, Pillar G, Gavriely N, Odeh M. Sublingual electrical stimulation of the tongue during wakefulness and sleep. Respir Physiol. 2001;127:217–26.
7. Johns MW. A new method for measuring daytime sleepiness: the Epworth sleepiness scale. Sleep. 1991;14:540–5.
8. Schwartz A, Bennett J, Smith P, et al. Therapeutic electrical stimulation of the hypoglossal nerve in obstructive sleep apnea. Arch Otolaryngol Head Neck Surg. 2001;127:1216–23.
9. Eastwood P, Barnes M, Walsh J, Maddison K, et al. Treating obstructive sleep apnea with hypoglossal nerve stimulation. Sleep. 2011;34:1479–86.
10. Van de Heyning P, Badr S, Baskin J, Bornemann M, et al. Implanted upper airway stimulation device for obstructive sleep apnea. Laryngoscope. 2012;122:1626–1633.
11. Mwenge GB, Rombaux P, Dury M, Lengele B, Rodenstein D. Targeted hypoglossal neurostimulation for obstructive sleep apnoea: a 1-year pilot study. Eur Respir J. 2013;41:360–7.
12. Vanderveken OM, Maurer JT, Hohenhorst W, Hamans E, Lin HS, Vroegop AV, Anders C, de Vries N, Van de Heyning PH. Evaluation of drug-induced sleep endoscopy as a patient selection tool for implanted upper airway stimulation for obstructive sleep apnea. J Clin Sleep Med. 2013;9(5):433–8.

Chapter 11
Robotic Setting

Mark A. D'Agostino, Gregory A. Grillone, and Federico Faedi

11.1 Introduction

There are a series of important steps that need to be taken in an organized and sequential fashion in order to perform a safe and successful transoral robotic surgical (TORS) procedure for obstructive sleep apnea [1]. The operating room setup includes the operating table, anesthesia cart, patient cart (robot), vision cart, instrument table, and surgeon's console. The positioning of each of these plays an important role in allowing safe and sufficient access to the patient, and allowing proper positioning of the robot to give the best possible visualization and access to the operative field. Proper personnel, instrumentation, patient positioning, and protection are of the utmost importance.

M.A. D'Agostino, M.D., F.A.C.S. (✉)
Department of Otolaryngology—Head & Neck Surgery, Middlesex Hospital, Middletown, CT, USA

Southern New England Ear, Nose and Throat Group, New Haven, CT, USA
e-mail: madago@comcast.net

G.A. Grillone, M.D., F.A.C.S.
Department of Otolaryngology, Boston University Medical Center, Boston, MA, USA
e-mail: Gregory.grillone@bmc.org

F. Faedi, M.S., Engineering
Head and Neck Department—ENT & Oral Surgery Unit, G.B. Morgagni—L. Pierantoni Hospital, Forli - Infermi Hospital, Faenza - ASL of Romagna, Italy
e-mail: faedi.federico@libero.it

© Springer International Publishing Switzerland 2016

C. Vicini et al. (eds.), *TransOral Robotic Surgery for Obstructive Sleep Apnea*,
DOI 10.1007/978-3-319-34040-1_11

11.2 Robotic System

Transoral robotic surgery is performed with the da Vinci® Surgical System (Intuitive Surgical, Sunnyvale, CA), which includes the robot (patient side cart) and the surgeon's operating console. Either the S HD or the Si da Vinci models are used. The newer Xi system may offer further advantages; however at the present time it is not approved for transoral cases. The system utilizes a high-definition camera available in both 0° and 30° (both available in 12 and 8 mm sizes). The camera offers a very clear high-definition 3-D image and provides up to 10× magnification, allowing for clear visualization in the oral cavity and easy visualization of vital structures such as nerves and vessels [2]. For transoral procedures, two 5 mm articulated instrument arms (Endo Wrist®) are used.

11.3 Surgeon's Console

The operating console should be off to the side or in a corner of the operating room. It should be located on the same side of the room as the head of the bed and operating assistant to allow free communication between the two and to allow quick access in the event of an emergency. The console offers the surgeon a high-definition 3-D image through stereoscopic eyepieces. Fingertip master controls allow full range of wrist and finger motion and translate these movements into precise movements of the surgical instruments loaded into the robotic arms. Foot pedals operate control of the cautery (monopolar or bipolar) and assist with control of the camera. A comfortable chair on wheels with back support and adjustable height should be available at the console for the surgeon. The console's settings are adjusted to the individual needs of the surgeon (i.e., height and angle of the monitor, height and position of the wrist rest) and the surgeon's preferences are stored in the console's memory for future cases.

11.4 Operating Room Setup

The operating room configuration for TORS in sleep apnea patients consists of the surgeon's operating console, the robot (patient side cart), the anesthesia cart, operating table, instrument cart, and the vision cart. The operating table is rotated 90–180° away from the anesthesia cart depending on the surgeon's preference. The author prefers to rotate the table approximately 130° away from anesthesia rather than a complete 180°. This rotation is necessary to allow complete access to the head of the bed and extension of the robotic arms over the patient's head. The anesthesia cart is at the foot of the bed or on the left side of the patient (depending on the amount of bed rotation), leaving the patient's right side free for docking of the robot. The surgical assistant sits at the head of the bed, and should be well trained in the operation of the robot including docking, undocking, and loading of the instruments. The surgical assistant is necessary to help with suctioning, retraction, hemostasis, and removal of specimen. The assistant is also the one to alert the surgeon of any problems or collisions with the robotic arms that may be out of the surgeon's view in the console. The surgeon needs to be notified immediately by the assistant if it is observed that one of the instruments is placing pressure on the dentition or any other structure. The vision cart consisting of the light source, image-processing equipment, monitor, and electrocautery unit is situated behind the assistant on the left side. Just to the right of the vision cart is a headlight to assist with placement of the gag, and a box of disposable gloves. The scrub nurse and instrument cart are located according to the different layouts of the operating room and according to the surgeon's preferences. The robot is docked along the right side of the bed at a slight angle of approximately 30°, paralleling the angle along the base of the operating table; this will vary based on the type of table used. If the robot is completely parallel to the bed it will be difficult to reach the surgical field with all three robotic arms. The operating console should be located off to the side or corner of the operating room on the same side as the surgical assistant. There needs to be a clear path between the operating console and the head of bed in the event of an emergency, to allow the surgeon quick access to the patient. Several monitors are positioned around the room to allow visualization for the entire OR team. One monitor is positioned just to the left of the patient for the seated surgical assistant to view; a second monitor is positioned so as to be viewed by the anesthesia team. A third monitor is attached to the side of the endoscopic tower for the scrub tech, circulating nurses, and any other observers in the room to view.

11.5 Patient Preparation

After induction of general anesthesia with nasotracheal or orotracheal intubation, the bed is rotated away from the anesthesia cart. Nasotracheal intubation allows a better exposure of the surgical field, but may not be practical if concurrent nasal surgery is to be performed. According to the surgeon preference it is possible to tape the pilot cuff of the endotracheal tube to the tube itself to avoid getting the robotic instruments caught and accidently dislodging the endotracheal tube during the procedure, since this is out of the surgeon's view in the console. If orotracheal intubation is used it is recommended that the anesthesiologist tape the tube to the corner of the lower lip on the left side, and tape downward as opposed to off to the side. This helps to align the natural curve of the tube in the posterior oral cavity in such a way to maximize exposure. Blood pressure cuff and IV are preferably placed on the left side and the patient's right arm is tucked to allow docking and full access with the robot. Protective goggles are placed over the eyes and dentition guards are placed over the maxillary and mandibular dentition (Fig. 11.1). A Goettingen® table support (Karl Storz) retractor holder is attached to the left side of the bed and is used to hook the mouth gag (Fig. 11.2). Alternatively an inexpensive Mayo instrument stand can be used to suspend the mouth gag with or without an extender (Dedo®)

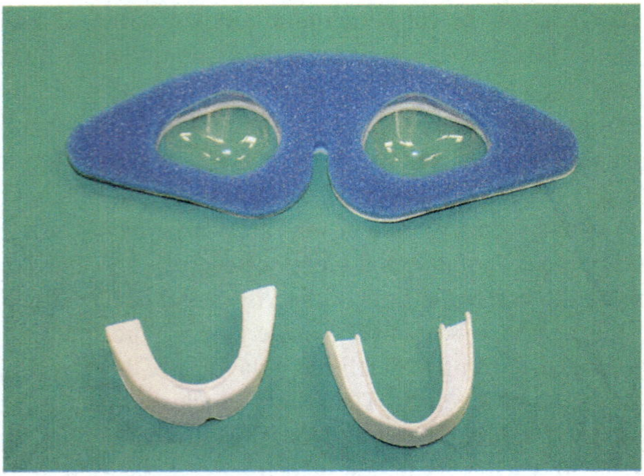

Fig. 11.1 Protective goggles can be placed over the eyes and dentition guards can be placed over the maxillary and mandibular dentition

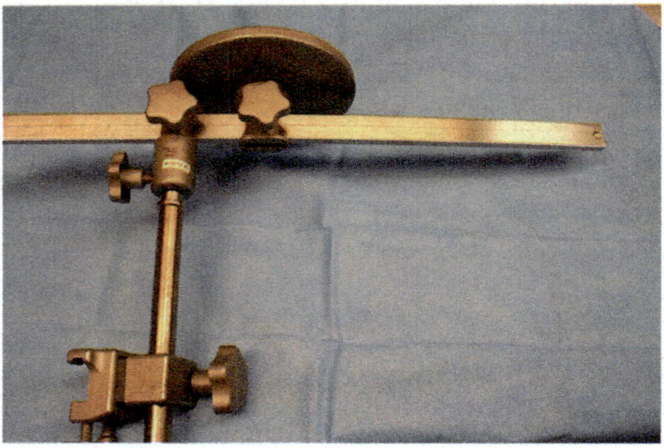

Fig. 11.2 Goettingen® table support (Karl Storz) retractor holder can be attached to the left side of the bed and used to hook the mouth gag

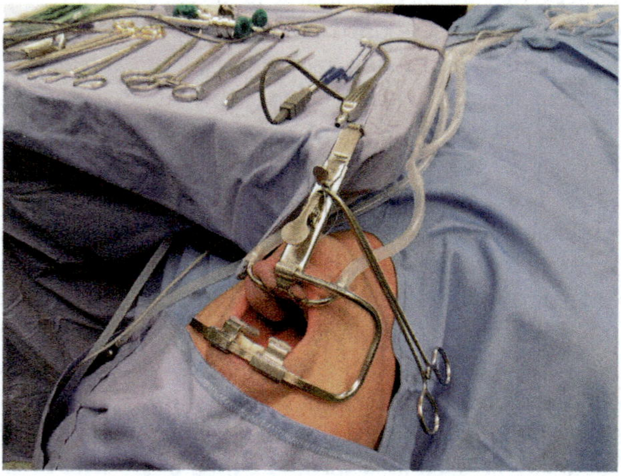

Fig. 11.3 Mayo instrument stand can be used to suspend the mouth gag with or without an extender (Dedo®)®

(Fig. 11.3). Three grounding pads are placed on the patient (one for the suction bovie ground, a second one for the robotic cautery ground, and a third pad to ground the robot). No shoulder roll is used. The patient's head is extended up and back as one would for a tonsillectomy ("sniffing position") [3]. Using a 0 silk stitch horizontal mattress suture is placed in the midline of the tongue to aid in retraction and placement of the gag. A hemostat is placed at the end of the stitch.

A number of different mouth gags are available. Many prefer the Feyh-Kastenbauer-Weinstein-O'Malley (FK-WO®) retractor (Olympus) which offers various sized tongue blades, attachable suction, and cheek retractors (Fig. 11.4). The author's preference is a Crowe-Davis® mouth gag (Bausch & Lomb/Storz) with Davis-Meyer® blades (Karl Storz) (Fig. 11.5). The Davis-Meyer blades are flat (with no indentation for endotracheal tube), have built-in suction ports, and come in ½ sizes [2, 4, 5]. Other available gags include Jennings® (Piling), and Dingman® (V. Mueller). The surgeon should hold off on placing the gag until the last moment before starting the case, to minimize pressure on the tongue and lingual nerve, thus avoiding a paresis of the lingual nerve. Once the gag is in place it is then hooked onto the Goettingen® retractor holder that is attached to the bed frame with the head slightly extended. The robot arms are then introduced into the oral cavity. The center arm with the camera is introduced first, bringing the operative field into full view, followed by the two side instrument arms. A Yankauer suction and a suction bovie are placed in an instrument holder attached to the drapes, for use by the surgical assistant, and a second suction setup is used to attach to the suction on the gag.

11.6 Robot Setup and Docking

The robot is draped with a sterile drape (Disposable Accessory Kit, 3-Arm Intuitive ref # 420290®) prior to the patient being brought into the operating room. The 3-D high-definition camera (0° and 30°, either 8 or 12 mm) is white balanced and calibrated using the target alignment guide (Intuitive®). When the patient is asleep and properly positioned the robot is brought up along the right side of the operating table.

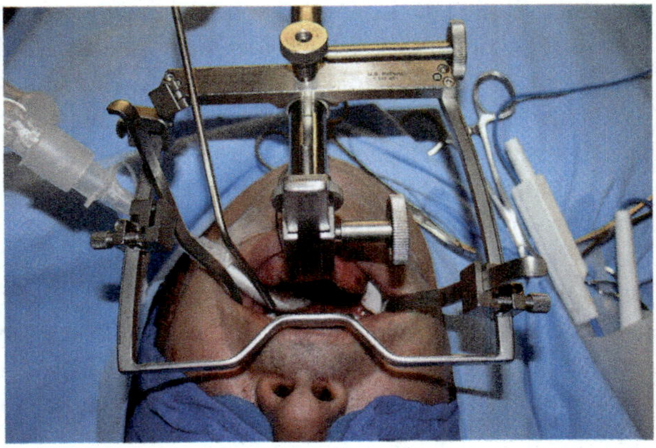

Fig. 11.4 Feyh-Kastenbauer-Weinstein-O'Malley (FK-WO®) retractor (Olympus) offers various sized tongue blades, attachable suction, and cheek retractors

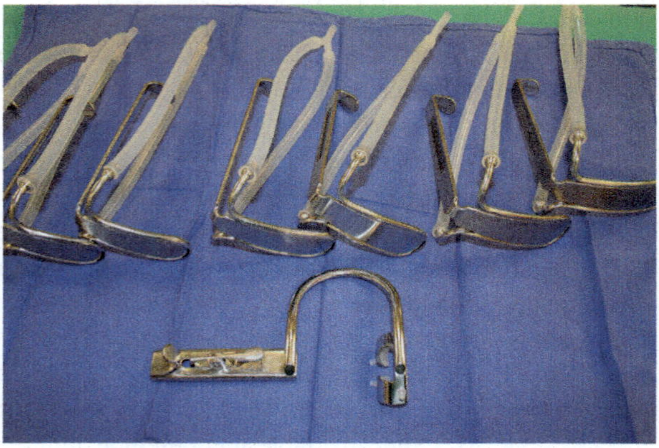

Fig. 11.5 Crowe-Davis® mouth gag (Bausch & Lomb/Storz) with Davis-Meyer® blades (Karl Storz)

The base of the robot is placed at an angle of approximately 30° from the base of the operating table, rather than parallel to it; this is to allow all three arms to reach over the patient's head and access the oral cavity without difficulty. The camera arm's joint should be positioned to the right to avoid collisions with the left instrument arm [4]. Make sure that there is adequate clearance between the instrument arms and the camera. The 5 mm flared cannulas (Intuitive PN420262®) are then positioned in the robotic arms and a grounding pad is attached to the cannula for the monopolar cautery instrument. The three robotic arms are loaded with the instruments of the surgeon's choice. The center arm is loaded with the 3-D high-definition scope (either a 0° or 30° high-definition scope, 8 or 12 mm). One may start with the 0° scope and switch to the 30° scope as the dissection proceeds. Otherwise, the procedure may be completely carried out by means of a 30° scope according to the surgeon's preference. The author prefers to use the 8 mm 30° scope for the entire case. The side arms (Arms #1 and #2) are loaded with instruments for cutting and retraction. Typically the 5 mm monopolar cautery with spatula tip (Intuitive PN 400160®) is used for cutting, and a 5 mm Maryland Dissector (Intuitive PN 400143/420143®) is used for retraction. Alternative options would be a 5 mm Schertel Grasper (Intuitive PN 400139/420139®) for retraction, or the 5Fr Introducer instrument (PN 400225/420143®) with a laser fiber for an alternative cutting device. At this point the mouth gag is inserted, opened, and hooked onto the Goettingen® retractor holder that is attached to the bed frame. The camera is then positioned into the midline of the oral cavity with the camera arm vertical (perpendicular to the patient) and as high up on the patient cart (robot) as possible to minimize collisions with the instrument arms. The cannula tip should be just inside the oral cavity at the level of the dentition and midway between the mandibular and maxillary dentition. Some prefer to have the cannula higher up, outside the oral cavity completely, to provide more space for the instrument arms and decrease the chance of collisions. Next the instrument arms are introduced one at a time. The tip of each instrument cannula should also be just inside the oral cavity with the majority of the cannula out of the oral cavity. The cannula can be positioned with a little tension on the commissure of the lips on each side to function as very mild buccal retraction.

The depth of the cannula insertion may be set in order to align the black ring at the level of the oral commissure (the black ring is the pivoting point of the arm, it does not move during any step of the surgery). Check to make sure that the joint of each instrument arm has clearance from the joint to the camera arm [4]. Next the pivotal axis of each instrument cannula is checked to make sure that it is at the level of the oral commissure or just outside of the oral cavity. Each instrument is then lowered through the cannula so that the tip is just past the camera allowing for visualization at the surgeon's console.

11.7 Instrument Table

The back instrument table should contain all the necessary instruments for the procedure and those necessary in the event of an emergency. Standard instruments include the oral gag and its accessories (i.e., various sized tongue blades), hemostats, DeBakey pickups, needle drivers, tonsillar hemostat, tonsil sponges, curved Allis, Herd pillar retractor, O- silk suture, the robotic cameras and instruments (5 mm Maryland dissector, monopolar cautery, etc.), vascular hemostatic clips, Tisseel® or Floseal® (Baxter Healthcare), and a bowl of saline and bulb syringe (in the event of an airway fire). The surgical assistant will need instruments to help retract the tongue; for this we have found a Freer, nerve root retractor, and the malleable suction monopolar cautery tip to be the most helpful. Specimen cups and an empty syringe (for quantifying the amount of tissue removed by volume displacement) should also be available on the instrument table.

References

1. Hoff P, D'Agostino M, Thaler E. Transoral robotic surgery in benign diseases including obstructive sleep apnea: safety and feasibility. Laryngoscope. 2015;125(5):1249–53.
2. Vicini C, Montevecchi F, Magnuson JS. Robotic surgery for obstructive sleep apnea. Curr Otorhinolaryngeal Rep. 2013;1:130–6.
3. Vicini C, Montevecchi F, Tenti G, Canzi P, Dallan I, Huntley T. Transoral robotic surgery: tongue base reduction and supraglottoplasty for obstructive sleep apnea. Oper Tech Otolaryngol. 2012;23(1):45–7.
4. O'Malley BW, Weinstein GS. da Vinci Tansoral Surgery Procedure Guide. Intuitive Surgical 2012; PN 871671.
5. D'Agostino MA. Transoral robotic partial glossectomy and supraglottoplasty for obstructive sleep apnea. Oper Tech Otolaryngol. 2015;26:211–5. published online 4 Aug 2015.

Chapter 12
Surgical Anatomy in Transoral Robotic Procedure: Basic Fundamentals

Iacopo Dallan, Lodovica Cristofani-Mencacci, Giovanni D'Agostino, Ermelinda Zeccardo, and Hesham Negm

12.1 Introduction

Transoral robotic procedures gained wide acceptance in the treatment of different lesions involving several sub-sites of the head and neck, with the oropharynx the most commonly addressed one (Fig. 12.1). The most evident consequence has been the need "to see" the anatomical structures from a new perspective, with a less important role played by the traditional, well-known, surgical landmarks. This "inside-out" vision must be well understood by those surgeons dealing with transoral robotic-assisted procedures (Fig. 12.2).

I. Dallan, M.D. (✉)
First ENT Unit, Azienda Ospedaliero-Universitaria Pisana, Via Paradisa, 2, 56126 Pisa, Italy

Head and Neck Surgery & Forensic Dissection Research Center (HNS & FDRC), Department of Biotechnology and Life Sciences (DBSV), University of Insubria, Varese, Italy
e-mail: iacopodallan@tiscali.it

L. Cristofani-Mencacci, M.D.
First ENT Unit, Azienda Ospedaliero-Universitaria Pisana, Via Paradisa, 2, 56126 Pisa, Italy
e-mail: lodovicacristofani@yahoo.it

G. D'Agostino, M.D.
Head and Neck Department—ENT & Oral Surgery Unit, G.B. Morgagni—L. Pierantoni Hospital, ASL of Romagna, Forlì, Italy

Infermi Hospital, ASL of Romagna, Faenza, Italy
e-mail: dago77@libero.it

E. Zeccardo, M.D.
Head and Neck Department—ENT & Oral Surgery Unit, G.B. Morgagni–L. Pierantoni Hospital, ASL of Romagna, Forlì, Italy

Infermi Hospital, ASL of Romagna, Faenza, Italy
e-mail: lindazeccardo@gmail.com

H. Negm, M.B.B.C.H., M.Sc., M.D.
Department of Otorhinolaryngology, Faculty of Medicine, Cairo University, Cairo, Egypt
e-mail: drnegment@hotmail.com

© Springer International Publishing Switzerland 2016

C. Vicini et al. (eds.), *TransOral Robotic Surgery for Obstructive Sleep Apnea*,
DOI 10.1007/978-3-319-34040-1_12

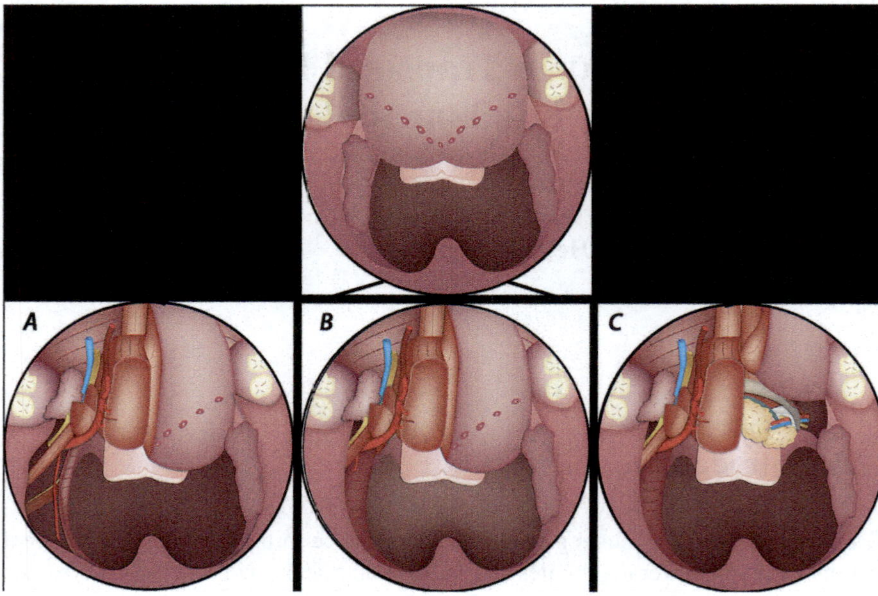

Fig. 12.1 Cartoon scheme showing potential applications of transoral robotic surgery. **a**—tongue base and parapharynx; **b**—tongue base; **c**—larynx (mainly supraglottic area) and hypopharynx

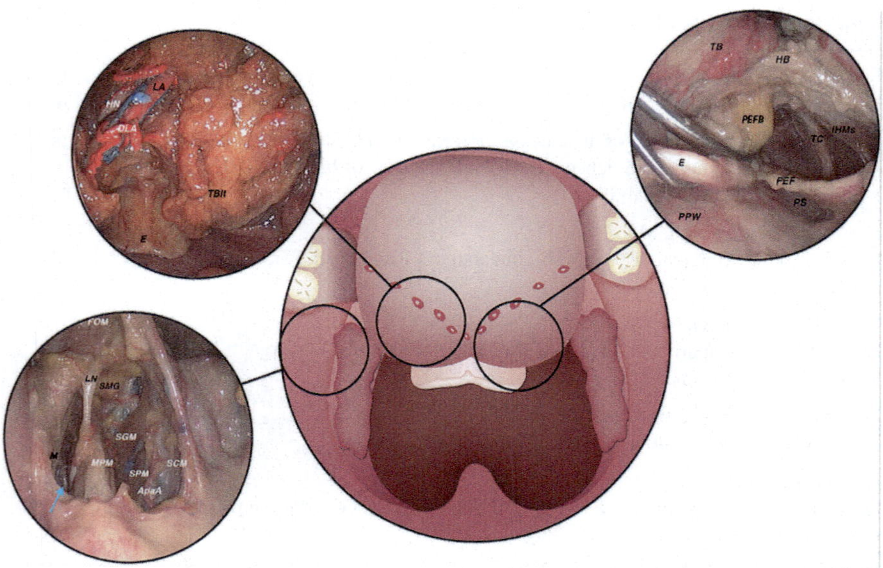

Fig. 12.2 Schematic pictures showing anatomical areas/regions manageable via transoral robotic surgery. *ApaA* ascending palatine artery, *DLA* dorsal lingual artery, *E* epiglottis, *FOM* floor of the mouth, *HN* hypoglossal nerve, *LA* lingual artery, *LN* lingual nerve, *M* mandible, *MPM* medial pterygoid muscle, *PEF* pharyngo-epiglottic fold, *PEFB* pre-epiglottic fat body, *PPW* posterior pharyngeal wall, *PS* piriform sinus, *SCM* superior constrictor muscle, *SGM* styloglossal muscle, *SMG* submandibular gland, *SPM* stylopharyngeal muscle, *TB* tongue base, *TBlt* tongue base lymphoid tissue, *TC* thyroid cartilage, *light-blue arrow* indicates inferior alveolar nerve

12.2 Oropharynx and Parapharyngeal Space

The oropharynx is the region of the pharynx between the soft palate and the epiglottis, and is continuous with the oral cavity anteriorly. It can be compared to a box opened anteriorly. Its limits are represented by: the palatine arches and palatine tonsils laterally; the posterior border of the soft palate superiorly; the dorsum of the tongue inferiorly; and the posterior pharyngeal wall posteriorly. The surface of the oropharynx is covered by stratified squamous epithelium. For didactic purpose the tonsillar region will be described in association with the parapharyngeal space. The tongue base will be discussed separately.

12.2.1 Palatine Tonsil, Lateral Pharyngeal Wall, and Parapharyngeal Space

The palatine tonsils are a paired lymphoid organ contained by the tonsillar capsule, a thin capsule originating from the pharyngobasilar fascia that covers the deep aspect of the tonsil. The fascia extends into the tonsil forming septa that carry nerves and blood vessels. The medial border of the tonsil is a free surface and contains folds and crypts. The tonsil is located in the tonsillar fossa, bordered anteriorly by the palatoglossus muscle and posteriorly by the palatopharyngeus muscle. The superior constrictor muscle (SCM) forms the majority of the lateral aspect of the tonsillar fossa and the inferior aspect of the fossa is comprised of the middle constrictor muscle (MCM). The glossopharyngeal nerve lies just deep to the SCM, and both the facial and lingual arteries can be very close to the inferior pole of the tonsil [1]. Furthermore, an abnormally long styloid process may extend into the tonsillar fossa in rare cases (4 %).

From a transoral perspective, the parapharyngeal space (PPS) lies lateral to the SCM. Within the fat of the PPS and deep to the SCM many nameless nerves and vessels can be found. On the lateral surface of the SCM, the *ascending palatine artery* (ApaA) and *ascending pharyngeal artery* (APA) can be found (Figs. 12.3 and 12.4). The ApaA is normally a branch of the facial artery while the APA is normally the smallest branch of the external carotid artery (ECA); The APA rarely arises from the occipital or the lingual artery. The lateral aspect of the PPS is formed by the medial pterygoid muscle (MPM), connecting the angle of the mandible with the inferior aspect of the pterygoid plates [2]. The lingual nerve runs in an anteroinferior direction between the body of the mandible and the MPM as it courses toward the floor of the mouth. Deep in the masticator space the inferior alveolar nerve can be identified, entering the vertical ramus of the mandible (Fig. 12.5). Medial to the MPM, the styloglossus muscle (SGM) and stylopharyngeus muscle (SPM) can be identified, both enveloped in a fascial system (styloid diaphragm). The styloid diaphragm appears as a thick fascia through which the anatomic elements of the retrostyloid space can be seen.

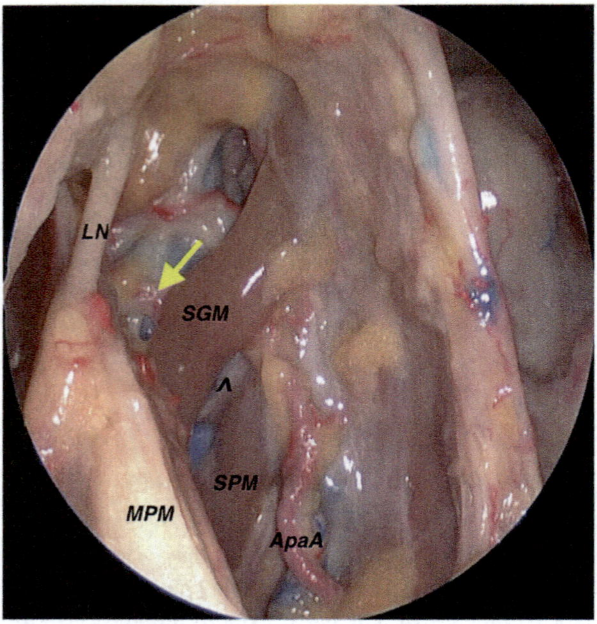

Fig. 12.3 Transpharyngeal window to the parapharyngeal space. The role of styloglossal and stylopharyngeal muscles is outlined. *ApaA* ascending palatine artery, *LN* lingual nerve, *MPM* medial pterygoid muscle, *SPM* styloglossal muscle, *black arrowhead* indicates glossopharyngeal nerve, *yellow arrow* indicates the origin of ApaA from the facial artery

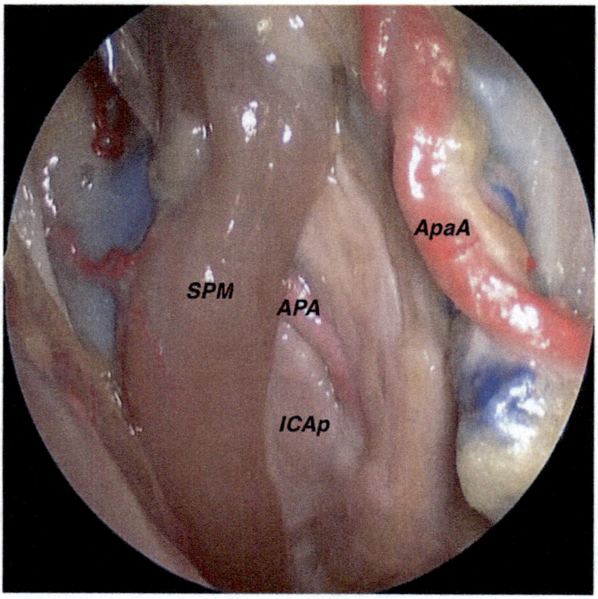

Fig. 12.4 Transpharyngeal window to the parapharyngeal space: close up vision showing the typical relationship between the ascending pharyngeal artery and the parapharyngeal portion of the internal carotid artery. *APA* ascending pharyngeal artery, *ApaA* ascending palatine artery, *ICAp* parapharyngeal portion of the internal carotid artery, *SPM* stylopharyngeal muscle

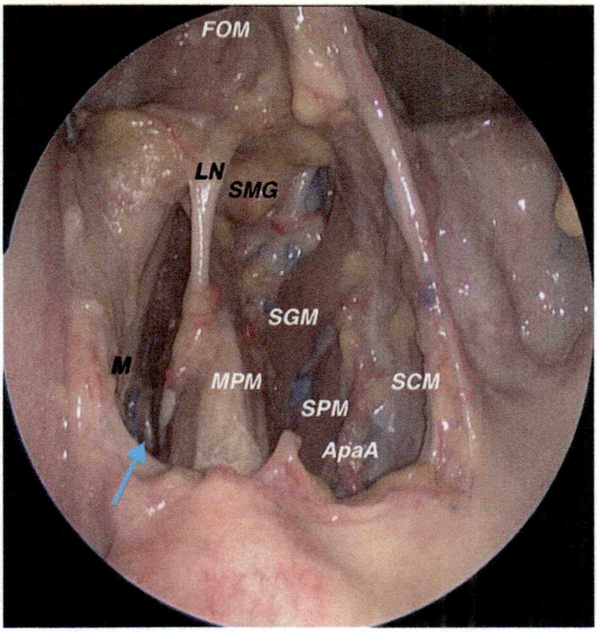

Fig. 12.5 Transpharyngeal window to parapharyngeal space: general overview. *ApaA* ascending palatine artery, *FOM* floor of the mouth, *LN* lingual nerve, *M* mandible, *MPM* medial pterygoid muscle, *SCM* superior constrictor muscle, *SGM* styloglossal muscle, *SMG* submandibular gland, *SPM* stylopharyngeal muscle, *light-blue arrow* indicates the inferior alveolar nerve entering the mandible

The SGM reaches the base of the tongue where it fuses with the inferior longitudinal and hyoglossus muscles. SPM is located more posterior with respect to SGM, and the glossopharyngeal nerve can be identified on the lateral surface of the SPM [2] (Fig. 12.3). The SPM is oriented in a more horizontal plane than the SGM. The deep lobe of the parotid gland can be visualized lateral to the styloid process.

Dissecting inferiorly in the PPS toward the floor of the mouth (Fig. 12.6) allows for identification of the facial artery and the lingual part of the submandibular gland, which lies above the mylohyoid muscle. It is sometimes possible to visualize the origin of the ascending palatine artery from the facial artery itself.

The bellies of the SGM and of the SPM represent a very important landmark to guide the identification of further anatomic elements and safe dissection in the PPS [2]. In the space between these muscles, in close relationship to the superior constrictor muscle, the so-called pharyngeal venous plexus, a complex venous network, can be visualized. This plexus should be well managed during lateral pharyngeal wall surgery in order to avoid post-operative bleeding. The ApaA and APA run a vertical course along the lateral surface of the superior constrictor muscle. Identification of the ascending pharyngeal artery can be considered a sentinel landmark for the parapharyngeal portion of the internal carotid artery [2]. Not infrequently, the APA and parapharyngeal portion of the internal carotid artery (ICAp) are covered by the bellies of SGM and SPM. Unfortunately, this relationship cannot be taken as a rule because the presence of looping or kinking of the ICAp. In such cases the artery lies in a more anterior plane with respect to the muscular bellies.

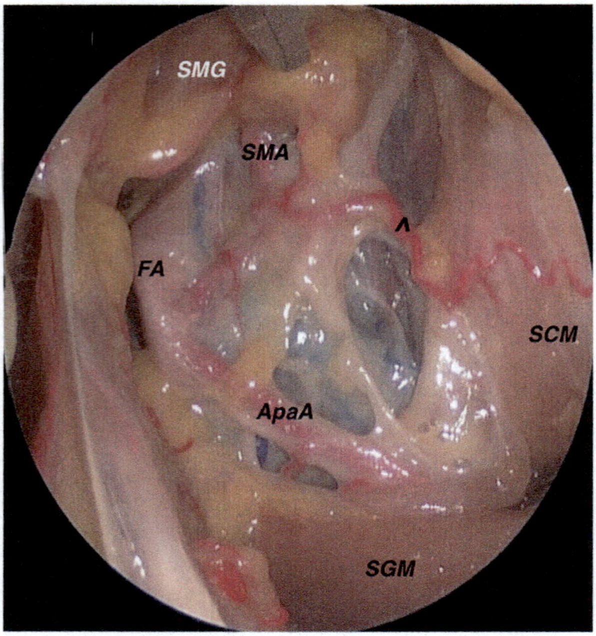

Fig. 12.6 Transpharyngeal window to parapharyngeal space: detail on the floor of the mouth. *ApaA* ascending palatine artery, *FA* facial artery, *SMA* submental artery, *SCM* superior constrictor muscle, *SGM* styloglossal muscle, *SMG* submandibular gland, *black arrowhead* indicates a facial artery branch for the tongue base

The ICAp lies lateral to the internal jugular vein (IJV). The external carotid artery (ECA) is normally located in the pre-styloid space, anterior and lateral to the styloid muscles. It is separated from ICAp by the SPM and SGM (Figs. 12.7 and 12.8).

Visualization of cranial nerve (CN) IX and X is difficult during transoral procedures. In the small angle between ICAp and IJV the initial extracranial portion of the lower cranial nerves can be seen. Their mutual relationship may be variable, but typically the glossopharyngeal nerve is the most medial, while the vagus nerve is consistently found in the posterior carotid-jugular angle. The accessory nerve usually curves rapidly backward in front of the IJV. The so-called pharyngeal plexus is a complex nerve plexus deriving from the anastomosis between the vagus nerve, the glossopharyngeal nerve, and the sympathetic cervical chain, and provides minor sensory and motor innervation to the muscles of the lateral pharyngeal wall. Medial and caudal to SGM, the greater cornu of the hyoid bone and the tendon of the digastric muscle can be identified. Caudal to the belly of the styloglossus muscle, the most important anatomic elements are the lingual artery and vein.

12.2.1.1 Blood Supply

The vascular supply of the tonsillar fossa and the lateral pharyngeal wall is based on the branches of the ECA. Arterial supply is given by:

- tonsillar branch (of facial artery) and ascending palatine artery, both branches of the facial artery;

- tonsillar branch of the dorsal lingual artery;
- tonsillar branch of the ascending pharyngeal artery;
- lesser palatine artery.

Most of these arteries enter the tonsil close to the inferior pole.

The *facial artery* is the fourth branch of ECA. It origins from ECA close to the lower border of the digastric muscle beneath the angle of the mandible. It runs, 5–8 mm deep to the stylohyoid and posterior belly of the digastric muscle, along with the lingual and ascending pharyngeal arteries. It may pass on or through the submandibular gland. Its tonsillar branch can run between, anterior, or posterior to the styloglossus muscles, with a high percentage of anatomic variability.

Surgical Considerations When performing radical tonsillectomy, the surgeon should consider that ECA branches might be very close to the superior constrictor and styloglossus muscles. Ligation of these terminal arteries can be performed both transorally and transcervically. The transcervical approach is considered by many to be safer and may be performed during staged neck dissection before radical tonsillectomy or base of tongue resection.

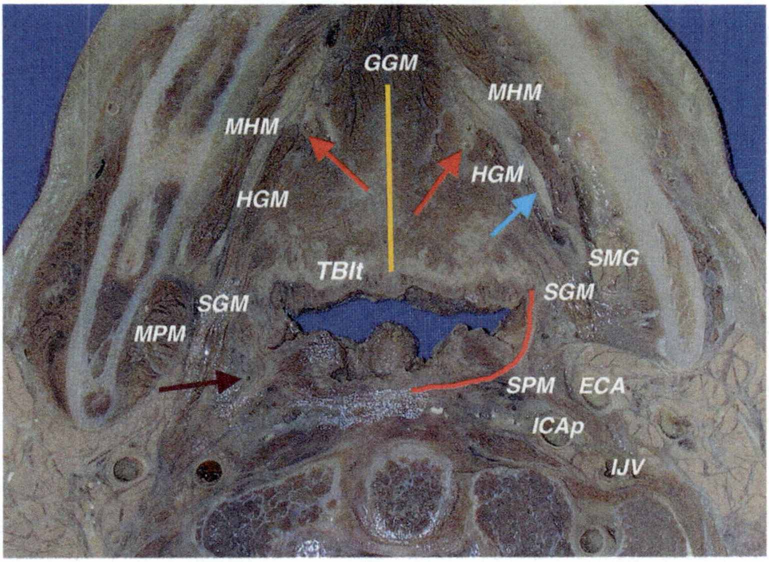

Fig. 12.7 Axial view of the parapharyngeal space. *ECA* external carotid artery, *GGM* genioglossal muscle, *HGM* hyoglossal muscle, *ICAp* parapharyngeal portion of the internal carotid artery, *IJV* internal jugular vein, *MHM* mylohyoid muscle, *MPM* medial pterygoid muscle, *SGM* styloglossal muscle, *SMG* submandibular gland, *SPM* stylopharyngeal muscle, *TBlt* tongue base lymphoid tissue, *purple arrow* indicates the ascending palatine artery, *red arrows* indicate lingual artery, *light-blue* arrow indicates the floor of the mouth portion of the lingual nerve, *yellow line* indicates the lingual septum, *light-red line* indicates the superior constrictor muscle

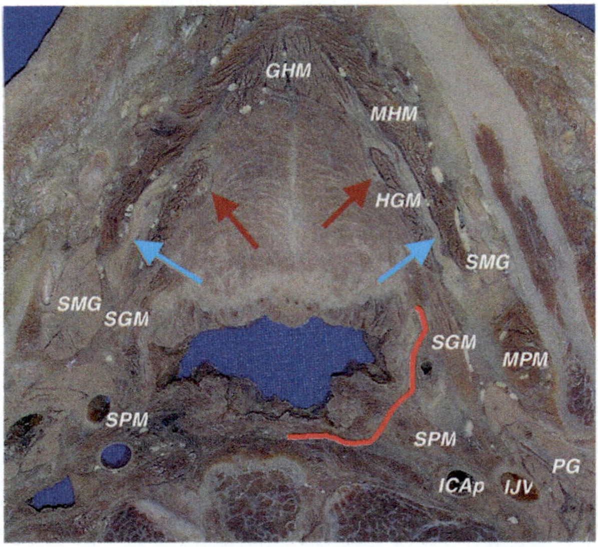

Fig. 12.8 Axial view of the parapharyngeal space. *GHM* geniohyoid muscle, *HGM* hyoglossal muscle, *ICAp* parapharyngeal portion of the internal carotid artery, *IJV* internal jugular vein, *SMG* submandibular gland, *MPM* medial pterygoid muscle, *PG* parotid gland, *SGM* styloglossal muscle, *SPM* stylopharyngeal muscle, *red arrow* indicate lingual arteries, *light-blue arrows* indicate floor of the mouth portion of the lingual nerve, *light-red line* indicates superior constrictor muscle

The *ascending palatine artery* originates from the facial artery in about 85 % of cases and in 70 % of cases it crosses the styloglossus muscle, before entering the pre-styloid space. In some cases it can originate directly from ECA or can course between SPM and SGM muscle before entering the PPS [3].

The *ascending pharyngeal artery* mainly originates from ECA. In few cases it may originate from ICA, the occipital artery, or may be absent [3]. This artery ascends vertically between the ICA and the lateral pharynx to the skull base along the longus capitis muscle.

The *external carotid artery* is located in the pre-styloid space; in more than 90 % of cases it is separated from ICA by the styloid diaphragm, pharyngeal venous plexus, and glossopharyngeal nerve. Rarely this artery bulges into the parapharyngeal fat between the styloglossus and stylopharyngeus muscles, adjacent to the pharyngeal constrictors. Surgery in the lateral pharyngeal space can result in injury to the ECA.

Knowledge of the anatomy of the *internal carotid artery* (ICA) and its variants is even more important. The course of the ICA in the parapharyngeal portion is usually straight and vertical as it courses toward the skull base [3, 4]. The ICAp is usually protected by the styloglossus and the stylopharyngeus muscles, which are medial and anterior to the vessel at the level of the oropharynx. According to Lim, the ICAp lies about 2.1 cm from the lateral pharyngeal wall at the level of the C2-C3 interspace [5]. Dissection lateral to the SCM may proceed safely in most cases; however, anatomical variants such as coiling or kinking of a tortuous ICAp do occur, and these anomalies may result in massive bleeding should inadvertent injury occur [6].

Surgical Considerations The presence of anatomical variants of ICA, if not recognized, may lead to ICA injury with potentially catastrophic complication. The critical role of the preoperative arterial-phase imaging is thus strongly advisable, so is the role of intraoperative Doppler.

12.2.1.2 Innervation

There are two important neural structures to be considered in TORS lateral pharyngeal wall surgery: the lingual nerve and the glossopharyngeal nerve (CN IX).

The *lingual nerve* is a branch of third branch of the trigeminal nerve (V3). From the posterior trunk of V3 it descends inferior and lateral to the medial pterygoid muscle and deep to the lateral pterygoid muscle, passing between the medial pterygoid and the vertical segment of the mandible. It then continues to run anteriorly and inferiorly, lateral to the styloglossus, and then the hyoglossus muscle until it reaches the floor of the mouth. The lingual nerve provides general sensation and taste to the anterior two-thirds of the tongue as well as parasympathetic innervation to the sublingual and the submandibular glands.

The *glossopharyngeal nerve* (CN IX) emerges from the skull base passing through the jugular foramen. It descends on the lateral side of the ICAp, medially to the styloid process, and between SPM and SGM. During its parapharyngeal course the nerve sends branches to the tonsil and to the posterior one-third of the tongue. The main trunk of the CN IX can be easily identified on the lateral surface of the SPM. Furthermore, it can be visualized at the intersection of the posterior tonsillar pillar with the base of tongue. The glossopharyngeal nerve provides sensation to the oropharynx, motor innervation to the SPM, and autonomic innervation to the parotid gland and carotid body.

Surgical Considerations The pharyngeal branch of CN IX may be very close to the tonsil fossa. Injury of this nerve, although rare, is possible during tonsillectomy and explains a possible post-operative dysgeusia.

12.2.2 Base of Tongue

The base of tongue is defined as the posterior part of the tongue, behind the circumvallate papillae. The epiglottis is connected to the tongue base by a median and two lateral glossoepiglottic folds. The depressions between these folds are called (pre-epiglottic) *valleculae*. Laterally, the tongue base is connected with the palatine tonsils by means of the glossotonsillar folds which is mainly derived from the palatoglossus muscle. Deep to the mucosa of the tongue base, and within the lymphoid tissue, a rich vascular arteriolar network is supplied by the paired dorsal lingual arteries. The amount of lymphoid tissue in the tongue base is highly variable; two distinct lingual tonsils are commonly visualized and are contiguous with the palatine tonsil at the glossotonsillar sulcus. Unlike the palatine tonsils, the lingual tonsils have no capsular bed, making complete removal difficult. Upon removal of the lingual tonsil tissue, tongue base muscle and the hyoid bone can be identified.

The tongue is composed of both intrinsic and extrinsic muscles. The intrinsic muscles are represented by the superior longitudinalis, inferior longitudinalis, transversus, and verticalis muscles. These muscles are bundles of interlacing fibers separated by connective tissue septa. The *midline lingual septum* is the strongest septum, and divides the tongue into two halves. The extrinsic muscles of the tongue include the genioglossus, hyoglossus, styloglossus, chondroglossus, and palatoglossus muscles. Except for the palatoglossus muscle, which is innervated by CN IX, all tongue muscles are innervated by the hypoglossal nerve (CN XII).

During tongue base dissection, the hyoid bone can easily be identified at the level of the glosso-epiglottic space (Fig. 12.9). The hyoid can be gently freed from its surrounding connections: anteriorly from the geniohyoid muscle which is inserted along the superior aspect of the hyoid body followed by the mylohyoid muscle; laterally, the middle constrictor inserts on to the hyoid at the level of the greater cornu. The medial portion of the tongue base is composed of the genioglossus muscle; however, it is not easily identified as a distinct muscle belly. In this area, where the genioglossus, mylohyoid, and geniohyoid muscles are in close approximation the area is commonly referred to as the "root of the tongue" [7]. The blood supply to the tongue is derived from the lingual artery which enters the tongue lateral and medial to the hyoglossus muscle.

The hypoglossal nerve and associated venae comitantes are located on the lateral aspect of the hyoglossus muscle [8] (Figs. 12.10 and 12.11). The lingual portion of the submandibular gland can be found further lateral and deep, lying above the mylohyoid muscle.

12.2.2.1 Blood Supply

The *lingual artery* is the second branch of the external carotid artery and originates inferior to the posterior belly of the digastric muscle and angle of the mandible. It runs anteriorly, close to the middle constrictor muscle, medial to the hypoglossal nerve, in close approximation to the greater cornu of the hyoid bone for a short distance before passing medial to the hyoglossus muscle; the artery gives off different branches to the tongue base (dorsal lingual arteries) and the body of the tongue. At this level (BOT) the artery lies on the lateral surface of the genioglossus muscle. At the anterior edge of the hyoglossus muscle the artery divides into its terminal branches, the *sublingual* and *deep lingual* arteries. The lingual vein forms from the

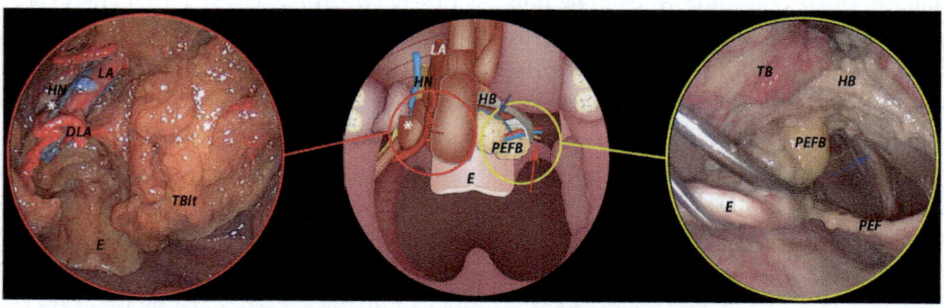

Fig. 12.9 Tongue base and supraglottic overview (transoral perspective). *DLA* dorsal lingual artery, *E* epiglottis, *HB* hyoid bone, *HN* hypoglossal nerve, *LA* lingual artery, *PEF* pharyngoepiglottic fold, *PEFB* pre epiglottic fat body, *TBlt* tongue base lymphoid tissue, *white asterisk* indicates hyoglossal muscle, *blue arrow* indicates thyroid cartilage, *red arrow* indicates superior laryngeal bundle

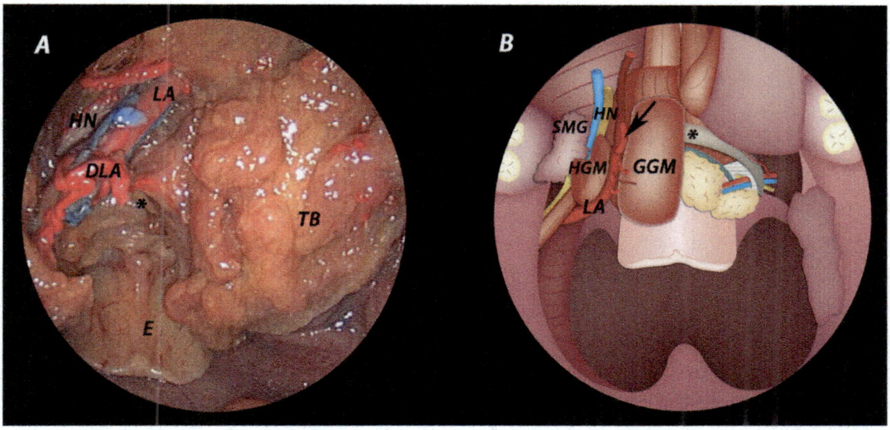

Fig. 12.10 Tongue base anatomy (transoral perspective). *DLA* dorsal lingual artery, *E* epiglottis, *GGM* genioglossal muscle, *HGM* hyoglossal muscle, *HN* hypoglossal nerve, *LA* lingual artery, *SMG* submandibular gland, *TB* tongue base, *black asterisk* indicates hyoid bone, *black arrow* indicates dorsal lingual artery

Fig. 12.11 Tongue base and inferior parapharyngeal regions (external perspective). *ABDM* anterior belly of the digastric muscle, *PBDM* posterior belly of the digastric muscle, *LA* lingual artery, *HGM* hyoglossal muscle, *MHM* mylohyoid muscle, *SGM* styloglossal muscle, *SHM* stylohyoid muscle, *SPM* stylopharyngeal muscle, *TB* tongue base, *IXcn* glossopharyngeal nerve, *XIIcn* hypoglossal nerve

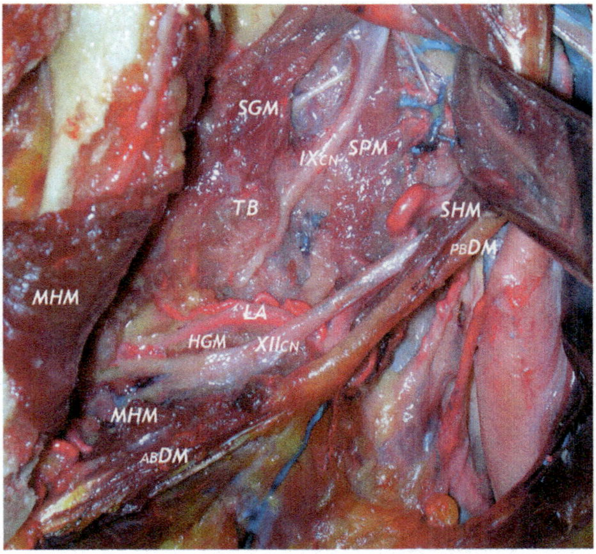

joining of small veins from the dorsum and side of the tongue. It accompanies the lingual artery and drains into the internal jugular or the facial veins.

Surgical Considerations Postoperative bleeding represents the most concerning complication related to TORS procedures. As a result of the numerous anastomoses that the lingual artery develops in its course, a transcervical ligation of the vessel is more effective than transoral management.

12.2.2.2 Innervation

The lingual nerve and the glossopharyngeal nerve have been described previously; they provide general sensation and taste to the anterior two-thirds (CN V) and posterior one-third (CN IX) of the tongue.

Motor innervation is provided by the *hypoglossal nerve* (CN XII). It emerges from the skull base through the hypoglossal foramen between the internal carotid artery and the internal jugular vein. It receives fibers from the first and second cervical nerves and gives rise to the *superior root of the ansa cervicalis*. The nerve turns anteriorly across the lateral surface of both the carotid vessels and around the sternocleidomastoid branch of the occipital artery above the hyoid bone. The hypoglossal nerve passes lateral to the hyoglossus muscle and over the greater cornu of the hyoid bone. It then continues above to the mylohyoid muscle and divides into terminal branches that run on the lateral surface of the genioglossus and enter the tongue musculature.

> **Surgical Considerations** Injury of the CN XII may occur during procedures that involve the area in which the nerve runs lateral to the hyoglossus muscle and above the hyoid bone. During transoral procedures these lesions are not common given the lateral and deep location of the nerve.

Tongue base reduction, as performed in TORS for OSAS cases, is designed to widen the oropharyngeal space by removing tissue (mostly lymphoid tissue). In this respect, it is of utmost importance to keep in mind that dissection in the midline is safe because no major neurovascular structures are present, while during lateral dissection the surgeon must consider the presence of the main trunk of the lingual artery, covered by the hyoglossal muscle [8]. Moreover, on the lateral surface of this muscle, lies the hypoglossal nerve and associated venae comitantes. The identification of the glossopharyngeal nerve is difficult in the tongue base because this nerve splits before entering the tongue base into small and variable tonsillar and lingual branches. The lingual branch enters the lateral tongue base so that, in the procedures necessitating a muscular tongue base resection, this branch is frequently cut.

12.3 Supraglottic Larynx

The first laryngeal structures visible with a transoral view include the epiglottis, the pharyngo-epiglottic folds and the aryepiglottic folds. As the depth of inspection proceeds inferiorly the arytenoid complex and the vocal cords are visualized. The epiglottis forms the anterior wall of the laryngeal aditus. The piriform sinuses are found lateral to the endolarynx and are bordered laterally by the inner surface of the thyroid cartilage and medially by the aryepiglottic fold.

The so-called *vestibule of the larynx* lies in the upper part of the larynx, extending from the aditus to the vestibular folds (false cords). The *vestibular folds*, also known as false vocal cords, are two folds of mucosa with a connective central core, that run from the thyroid cartilage anteriorly, to the bodies of the arytenoid cartilages posteriorly. Finally, the *ventricle of Morgagni*, is formed by lateral extensions of the mucosa above the true cords between the vestibular and the vocal cords. At the anterior end of the ventricle, under the vestibular folds, the *laryngeal saccule* (also named *appendix of the ventricle*), a diverticulum extends superiorly between the vestibular folds and the inner surface of the thyroid cartilage, can be dissected and visualized.

The tongue base (*pharyngeal tongue*) is "attached" to the supraglottic epiglottis by means of *glosso-epiglottic folds*, one median and two laterally (pharyngo-epiglottic folds). The epiglottis is directed upward and backward and lies in the upper portion of the larynx behind the tongue base and the hyoid bone, bordering the *pre-epiglottic space* posteriorly. The thyrohyoid membrane and thyroid cartilage border this space anteriorly, while the hyoid bone, the thyro-epiglottic ligament and valleculae form the superior border. Laterally the pre-epiglottic space is defined by the *paraglottic spaces*, which are confluent with it anteriorly. The pre-epiglottic space is occupied mainly by fat and areolar tissue. The thyrohyoid, sternohyoid, and omohyoid muscles lie anterior to the thyrohyoid membrane. A bursa is present between the upper portion of the thyrohyoid membrane and the body of the hyoid bone, increasing the mobility of the system.

The primary supporting structures of the larynx are the hyoid bone, and the thyroid and cricoid cartilages. The role of the hyoid bone is to allow movement of the larynx during swallowing and serves as an attachment point for the suprahyoid and infrahyoid muscles and stylohyoid ligament. The hyoid bone is connected to the epiglottis by the hyo-epiglottic ligament and to the pharyngeal wall by means of pharyngo-epiglottic folds. These folds are derived of mucosa. Dissection through the vallecula and pharyngo-epiglottic folds from above allows for identification of the hyoid bone (Fig. 12.12). The inferior part of the superior constrictor muscle arises from the lateral part of the root of the tongue while the middle constrictor

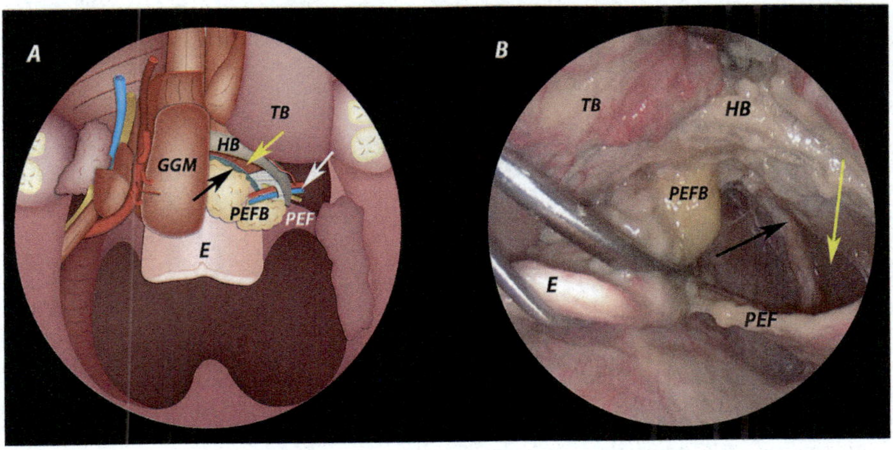

Fig. 12.12 Supraglottic anatomy (transoral perspective). *E* epiglottis, *GGM* genioglossal muscle, *HB* hyoid bone, *PEF* pharyngoepiglottic fold, *PEFB* pre epiglottic fat body, *TB* tongue base, *white arrow* indicates superior laryngeal bundle, *yellow arrow* indicates infrahyoid muscles, *black arrow* indicates thyroid cartilage

muscle is attached to the hyoid bone (at the level of the greater and lesser cornu); the hyoid bone lies medial to the middle constrictor. During transoral dissection in this area, the fibers of middle constrictor muscle are identified and transected. Lateral to the greater cornu of the hyoid bone the digastric muscle with its tendon can be visualized, as well as the stylohyoid muscle. The *bucco-pharyngeal gap* is an anatomical space defined by the superior constrictor, middle constrictor and mylohyoid muscles. This space transmits the lingual artery and nerve, the hypoglossal and glosso-pharyngeal nerves, as well as the styloglossus and hyoglossus muscles. At the level of the vallecular area within the glosso-epiglottic fold branches of the lingual artery can be identified, and should be managed. The superior laryngeal neurovascular bundle lies close to the hyoid bone and enters the larynx through the thyrohyoid membrane just inferior and anterior to the greater cornu of the hyoid bone. The superior laryngeal artery (SLA) accompanies the internal branch of superior laryngeal nerve (SLNib). In most cases the superior laryngeal vein accompanies the artery and the nerve; however, it may be absent in some patients. During transoral dissection the SLA can be easily identified in the pharyngo-epiglottic fold. Usually the artery passes inferiorly in the submucosa of the lateral wall of the piriform sinus as it courses toward the floor of the sinus itself (Fig. 12.13). The branches

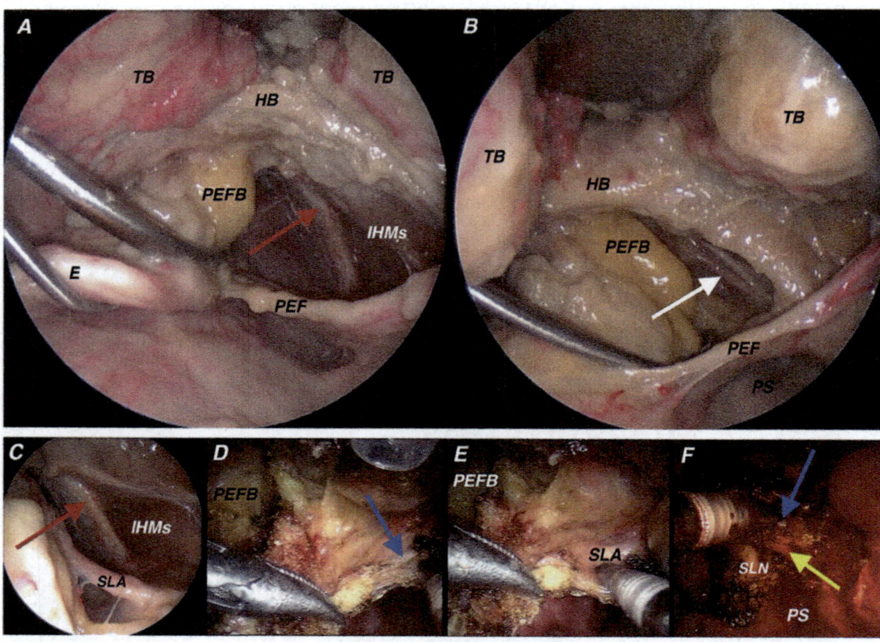

Fig. 12.13 Supraglottic anatomy (transoral perspective). *E* epiglottis, *HB* hyoid bone, *IHMs* infrahyoid muscles, *PEFB* pre epiglottic fat body, *PS* piriform sinus, *SLA* superior laryngeal artery, *SLN* superior laryngeal nerve (external branch), *TB* tongue base, *blue arrow* indicates superior laryngeal vein, *yellow arrow* indicates superior laryngeal nerve, *red arrow* indicates thyroid cartilage, *white arrow* indicates superior laryngeal artery

of SLA that are significant during supraglottic laryngectomy are the *superior* and *anterior* branches. The superior branch of the SLA runs along the aryepiglottic fold to the epiglottis, while the inferior branch of the SLA runs from its origin toward the superior margin of thyroid cartilage [9]. The superior branch supplies the laryngeal epiglottis and forms an anastomotic network with the *dorsal lingual arteries* in the vallecular region and lingual epiglottis [10] or with the *suprahyoid branch* of the lingual artery [11].

The vascular supply of the supraglottis includes dorsal branches of the lingual artery and the SLA. The dorsal lingual artery supplies the region of the vallecular area e lingual epiglottis [12].

Surgical Considerations The epiglottic cartilage has small perforations that contain mucous glands. These fenestrations may act as a route of entry for carcinoma into the pre-epiglottic space.

The major cartilages, ligaments, and membranes of the larynx form adipose filled spaces: the *pre-epiglottic*, *paraglottic*, and *subglottic* spaces. The *pre-epiglottic space* is anterior to the epiglottis and is bound by the thyroid cartilage and thyrohyoid membrane anteriorly, the median thyro-epiglottic ligament and vallecula superiorly, and the anterior surface of the epiglottic cartilage and the petiole posteriorly. This space is continuous with the paraglottic space laterally. The *paraglottic space* is a paired space bound by the inner perichondrium of the thyroid cartilage, conus elasticus, and quadrangular membrane anterolaterally, the laryngeal ventricle medially, and the piriform sinus mucosa posteriorly. The *subglottic space* boundaries are given by the vocal cord superiorly and by the conus elasticus superolaterally.

12.3.1 Blood Supply

The *superior laryngeal artery* (SLA) provides the dominant blood supply to the supraglottic larynx. It originates from the superior thyroid artery, near the superior pole of the thyroid gland. In about 30 % of cases it may arise directly from the external carotid artery. From its origin this artery passes horizontally across the posterior portion of the thyrohyoid membrane along with the internal branch of the superior laryngeal nerve, and pierces the membrane close to the nerve to enter the larynx. Here it travels within the pharyngo-epiglottic fold and divides into several branches. Up to five branches of the SLA have been described [9]. The most relevant branches to consider in TORS supraglottic procedures, are the *superior* and *anterior* branches of the SLA. The superior branch is the most superficial, in a craniocaudal orientation, and courses across the upper aspect of the piriform sinus to supply the epiglottis and the vallecular region. It forms an anastomotic network with dorsal branches of the lingual artery in the vallecula and the lingual epiglottis [10]. The anterior branch supplies the laryngeal ventricle, and can be identified inferiorly along the thyrohyoid membrane in the pre-epiglottic space [12]; this branch in fact runs from its origin toward the superior border of the thyroid cartilage [9]. A variant of SLA, the so-called *aberrant superior laryngeal artery* [13], enters the larynx through a thyroid foramen, located in the posterior part of the thyroid cartilage lamina.

Surgical Considerations Intraoperative vascular control should be obtained via ligation of the main trunk of the SLA. This vessel can be easily identified at the level of the pharyngo-epiglottic fold. The superior laryngeal vein runs parallel to SLA and drains into the superior thyroid vein.

12.3.2 Innervation

The superior laryngeal nerve is responsible of the innervation of this region. It originates from the inferior ganglion (nodose) of the vagus nerve. It runs medial to both the internal and external carotid arteries and divides into a small external and a large internal branch. The external branch gives a branch to the inferior constrictor muscle and supplies the cricothyroid muscle, usually lying very close to the superior thyroid artery. The internal branch travels along with SLA and pierces the thyrohyoid membrane. It then divides into a few branches (usually 2–3). The upper branches provide sensation to mucosa of the epiglottis, vallecula, vestibule and false vocal folds. The lower branch provides sensation to mucosa below the vestibule and the mucosa of the pyriform sinus. It also provides motor innervation, along with the recurrent laryngeal nerve, to the inter-arytenoid muscles. Preserving the inferior/lower branch during surgical dissection allows for sparing of mucosal sensory innervation of both the hypopharynx and larynx below the vestibule, and motor innervation of the inter-arytenoid musculature which helps to preserve the cough reflex.

12.4 Conclusions

A sound knowledge of anatomy has always been and remains fundamental to the performance of safe and effective surgery. Surgical anatomy has traditionally been taught from an "outside-in" perspective; however, as surgical approaches have evolved there are different ways to visualize these structures. In transoral robotic procedures, historical external landmarks have less importance, and "new" landmarks and approaches need to be identified and described from an "inside-out" orientation. In this chapter we try to offer a step-by-step, logical approach to the surgical anatomy of these critical areas from a transoral perspective, with commentary on critical elements relevant to the transoral surgeon.

References

1. Janfaza P, Nadol Jr JB, Galla RJ, et al. Surgical anatomy of the head and neck. Philadelphia, PA: Lippincott Williams & Wilkins; 2001.
2. Dallan I, Seccia V, Muscatello L, et al. Transoral endoscopic anatomy of the parapharyngeal space: a step-by-step logical approach with surgical considerations. Head Neck. 2011;33(4):557–61.
3. Wang C, Kundaria S, Fernandez-Miranda J, et al. A description of arterial variants in the transoral approach to parapharyngeal space. Clin Anat. 2014;27:1016–22.
4. Ozgur Z, Celik S, Govsa F, et al. A study of the course of the internal carotid artery in the parapharyngeal space and its clinical importance. Eur Arch Otorhinolaryngol. 2007;264:1483–9.
5. Lim CM, Metha V, Chai R, et al. Transoral anatomy of the tonsillar fossa and lateral pharyngeal wall: anatomic dissection with radiographic and clinical correlation. Laryngoscope. 2013;123:3021–5.
6. Vega J, Gervas C, Vega-Hazas G, Barrera C, Biurrun C. Internal carotid artery transposition: another cause of widening of the retropharyngeal space. Eur Radiol. 1999;9(2):347–8.
7. Moore EJ, Janus J, Kasperbauer J. Transoral robotic surgery of the oropharynx: clinical and anatomic considerations. Clin Anat. 2012;25:135–41.
8. Dallan I, Seccia V, Faggioni L, et al. Anatomical landmarks for transoral robotic tongue base surgery: comparison between endoscopic, external and radiological perspective. Surg Radiol Anat. 2013;35(1):3–10.
9. Rusu MC, Nimigean V, Banu MA, et al. The morphology and topography of the superior laryngeal artery. Surg Radiol Anat. 2007;29:653–60.
10. Imanishi N, Kondoh T, Kishi K, et al. Angiographic study of the superior laryngeal artery. Okajimas Folia Anat Jpn. 2009;86:61–5.
11. Yarlagadda BB, Grillone GA. Anatomic considerations in transoral robotic surgery. In: Grillone GA, Jalisi S, editors. Robotic surgery of the head and neck: a comprehensive guide. New York: Springer; 2015. p. 13–27.
12. Goyal N, Yoo F, Setabutr D, et al. Surgical anatomy of the supraglottic larynx using the da Vinci robot. Head Neck. 2014;36:1126–31.
13. Liu JL, Liang CY, Xiang T, et al. Aberrant branch of the superior laryngeal artery passing through the thyroid foramen. Clin Anat. 2007;20:256–9.

Chapter 13
Transoral Robotic Surgery for Obstructive Sleep Apnea Syndrome: An Anesthetist's Point of View

Ruggero Massimo Corso, Davide Cattano, and Nabil Abdelhamid Shallik

13.1 Introduction

A recent meta-analysis concluded that OSA patients who undergo noncardiac surgery have a higher rate of desaturation in the postoperative phase, respiratory failure, cardiac events, and unplanned transferals to intensive care compared to patients unaffected by OSA [1]. Postoperative complications are caused by the interaction between anesthetic agents, as well as sedatives and analgesic narcotics, and the pharyngeal muscular tone and reawakening response to hypoxia characteristics of patients affected by OSA; being predisposed to upper airway collapse in natural sleep, OSA patients are more sensitive to the effects of anesthetics and sedatives and may develop respiratory complications in the postoperative period. Most complications occur during the first 24–48 h in the postoperative phase. At a later stage (after a week), complications are mainly due to a rebound of rapid eye movement (REM) in sleep caused by the administering of high doses of opioids in the postoperative phase which suppress REM, causing sleep deprivation [2]. Cardiovascular stimulation by hypoventilation and acidosis, sympathetic activation, and hypoxia could also determine cardiovascular events. Various authors have suggested therapeutic clinical actions or have drafted recommendations to this aim [3, 4].

R.M. Corso, M.D. (✉)
Emergency Department, Anesthesia and Intensive Care Section, G.B. Morgagni—L. Pierantoni Hospital, Forlì, Italy
e-mail: rmcorso@gmail.com

D. Cattano, M.D., Ph.D.
UTH Medical School at Houston, Houston, TX, USA
e-mail: davide.cattano@uth.tmc.edu

N.A. Shallik, M.B., Ch.B., M.Sc., M.D.
Anesthesia, ICU and Perioperative Medicine Department, Hamad Medical Corporation, Doha, Qatar
e-mail: nabilsholik66@hotmail.com; nshallik@hamad.qa

© Springer International Publishing Switzerland 2016

C. Vicini et al. (eds.), *TransOral Robotic Surgery for Obstructive Sleep Apnea*, DOI 10.1007/978-3-319-34040-1_13

13.2 Preoperative Evaluation

The preoperative evaluation and medical optimization of the patient presenting for TORS procedures are key elements for the anesthesiologists and surgeons. Every preoperative evaluation should include (1) American Society of Anesthesiologists (ASA) physical status score; (2) planned anesthetic strategy {e.g., general, Monitored Anaesthesia Care (MAC) or regional}; (3) airway management strategy {awake fiber-optic intubation, video laryngoscopy (VL), direct laryngoscopy (DL), tracheostomy}; (4) indication for special monitoring (e.g., arterial catheter, central line); (5) likely need for blood products; and (6) indication for postoperative critical care management. Preoperative evaluation should be carried out with sufficient time before the scheduled procedure to allow for the implementation of any advisable preoperative intervention aimed at improving patient outcome. The reader is referred to the recent pertinent guidelines for further discussion [5].

13.3 Airway Management

Difficult airway management, combining difficult mask as well as difficult tracheal intubation, may be common in OSA patients [6, 7]. Airway strategies also need to be tailored considering that morbid obesity is often associated with severe OSA.

13.3.1 Optimizing Preoxygenation, Positioning (Safety Apnea Rescue Time)

The correct positioning of the patient is perhaps the most important element to ensure the success of airway control. A 25° head-up and reverse Trendelenburg positions increase the duration of apnea without arterial desaturation allowing more time for tracheal intubation. The "ramped" position achieved by the horizontal alignment of the sternal notch with the external auditory meatus using folded blankets or commercially available pillows under the upper body, shoulders, and head facilitates the direct laryngoscopy [8]. It is also important to carry out preoxygenation to avoid hypoxemia after induction of general anesthesia using positive airway pressure, supplemental nasopharyngeal oxygen insufflation, and noninvasive ventilation (NIV). Overall the goal is to provide an effective oxygenation that would last for a considerable time (3–5 min) in the event that a difficult airway occurs (safety apnea rescue time), resulting in a sustained period of hypoventilation, and before severe desaturation (oxygen saturation less than 90 %) occurs.

13.3.2 Airway Management Plans

The key to safely manage the airway in the OSA patient lies in the ability to predict difficulties and have communicated with the operating room team a strategy that includes multiple exit routes if needed. The multivariate risk index developed by El-Ganzouri and coworker [9] involves the analysis of seven parameters commonly performed during the preoperative evaluation and includes a history of difficult airway. Each variable is assigned a score (from 0 to 1); a score ≥4 has a high sensitivity for predicting a difficult tracheal intubation (DI) (Table 13.1). In a study by Corso et al. [10], El Ganzouri Risk Index (EGRI) has proven to work both in the prediction of DI and difficult mask ventilation (DMV); in this way the operator with a single bedside screening test is able to assign a red flag to selected cases, activating a specific clinical path in the busy operating room theater. Moreover Cortellazzi et al. [11] showed that the EGRI predictive test may acquire good accuracy when video laryngoscopy improves visualization of laryngeal structures in comparison to direct laryngoscopy. They suggested an algorithm based on the decision rule derived by an EGRI of 7 for every patient undergoing general anesthesia and routinely intubated with GlideScope® video laryngoscope. Figure 13.1 shows our strategy.

13.3.3 EGRI < 7: Direct Laryngoscopy Versus Video Laryngoscopy—Backup Supraglottic Airway Devices

Direct laryngoscopy can be aided by the use of a gum elastic bougie or an intubating malleable stylet, when suboptimal glottic views are obtained. Recently video laryngoscopy has definitely won its place in clinical practice. Avoiding the need to align oral and pharyngeal axes, video laryngoscopes (VLs) provide clear visualization and reliable intubation in patients with a difficult airway. Several studies have shown that video laryngoscopy improves intubation condition in morbidly obese patients [12].

Table 13.1 The multivariate risk index developed by El-Ganzouri

Composition of the El-Ganzouri and Colleagues' Multivariate Risk Index (EGRI)			
Variable/score	0	1	2
Interincisor gap	≥4 cm	<4 cm	
Thyromental distance	≥6.5 cm	6.0–6.5 cm	<6 cm
Modified Mallampati class	I	II	III, IV
Neck movement	>90°	80–90°	<80°
Ability to prognath	Yes	No	
Body weight	<90 kg	90–110 kg	>110 kg
History of DI	None	Questionable	Definite

DI: Difficult intubation, total EGRI Score

≥4: Difficult intubation predicted

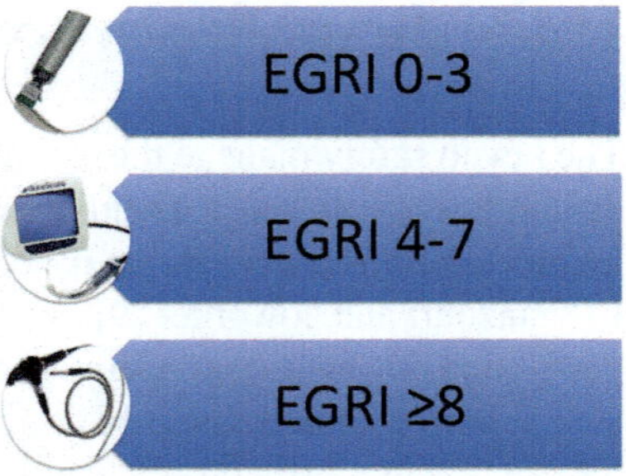

Fig. 13.1 Strategy of intubation at the Morgagni-Pierantoni Hospital based on the decision rule derived by EGRI for every patient undergoing general anesthesia

It should be kept in mind that although VLs improve visualization of the glottis, this is usually at the expense of prolonged tracheal intubation times and does not necessarily translate into easier intubation. Today, no single video laryngoscope has shown superiority for use in the obese patient and research to identify predictive factors of difficult video laryngoscopy is just beginning (Fig. 13.2). VLs can also be effectively used in awake intubation techniques. In the anesthetized patient, oral fiber-optic intubation may be difficult due to the collapse of the upper airway soft tissue: Supraglottic Airway Devices (SADs) (Fig. 13.3) can act as conduits to maintain an open airway and access to the laryngeal inlet. An endotracheal tube may be guided over a bronchoscope (Seldinger technique) through the SAD or an Aintree Intubating Catheter (Cook Critical Care, Bloomington, IN, USA) may be advanced over the bronchoscope into the trachea through the SAD. The fiberscope and SAD are then removed leaving the intubating catheter in situ to act as a "guidewire" device for endotracheal tube.

13.3.4 EGRI ≥ 8: Awake Fiber-Optic Intubation—Backup Supraglottic Airway Devices

Facing a predicted difficult airway, an awake fiber-optic intubation (AFOI) is recommended. Critical to the success of the technique is topical anesthesia with lidocaine and sedation. Among drugs used for sedation remifentanil target-controlled infusion (TCI) appears to provide better conditions for AFOI when compared with propofol® TCI in normal-weight patients. Dexmedetomidine is another option providing favorable intubation conditions during AFOI, without respiratory depression and airway obstruction. However, evidence about the optimal TCI sedation technique for AFOI in obese patients is lacking. Awake tracheal intubation using video laryngoscopy has emerged as a substitute for awake flexible fiber optic. Different devices and techniques can be combined, based on proper topical local anesthesia using specific devices (i.e., see the utilization of the D blade CMAC system, MAD atomizer, and topical anesthesia in different awake laryngoscopy/intubation scenarios).

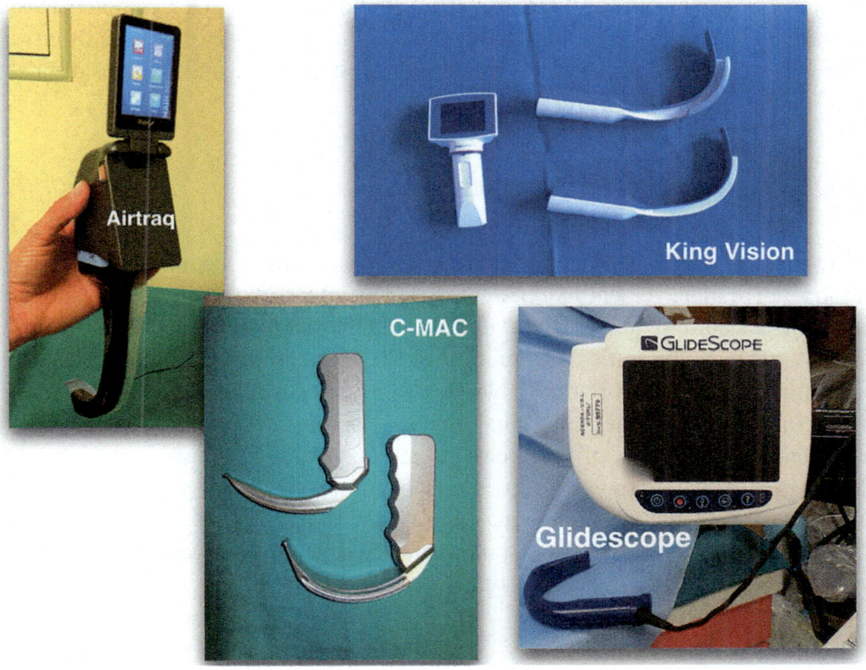

Fig. 13.2 Different types of video laryngoscopes

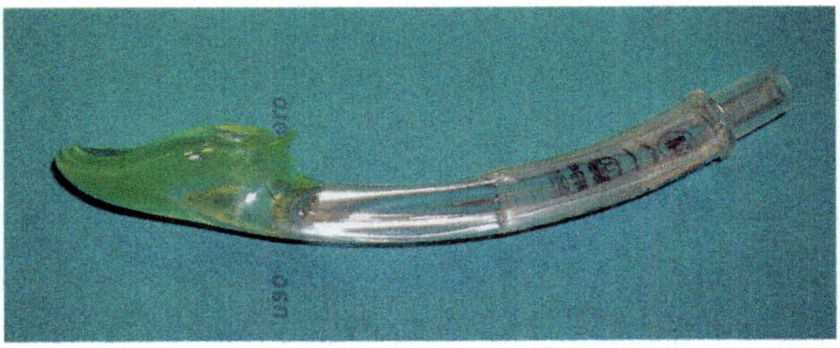

Fig. 13.3 The i-gel® is a second-generation supraglottic airway device used by one of the authors (RMC) in his department)

13.3.5 Safe Extubation

It has long been known that many airway-related complications occur at the time of tracheal extubation resulting in significant morbidity and mortality. In order to minimize risk to patients during tracheal extubation, a stepwise approach has been suggested by the Difficult Airway Society guidelines (DAS) [13]. Risk stratification of patients for high or low risk of complication during extubation is essential: morbidly obese and sleep apnea patients are regarded as high-risk category, and a set of specific recommendations are suggested focused on awake tracheal extubation. The importance of logistic factors is stressed including the selection of the operating room as the location for extubation and the presence of skilled assistance, equipment, and monitoring. The DAS guidelines also underline the importance of the use of airway exchange catheters in patients for whom tracheal re-intubation is likely to be difficult.

13.4 Intraoperative Management

There is no evidence to support recommendations for more aggressive or invasive intraoperative management in OSA patients. The intensity of monitoring should be established according to the nature of the scheduled surgical operation and the presence of other comorbidities. Monitoring for TORS includes standard ASA guidelines. In addition invasive arterial blood monitoring, Bispectral Index monitoring® (BIS), and neuromuscular monitoring can be performed on an individual basis. There is evidence that many anesthetic agents cause exaggerated responses in patients with sleep apnea. All common anaesthetics may blunt the tone of the pharyngeal musculature that acts to maintain airway patency. Anesthesia techniques using shorter acting drugs are attractive because a more rapid return to baseline respiratory function would be expected when shorter acting drugs are employed [14].

13.4.1 Mechanical Ventilation

Many clinical studies have attempted to find an optimal ventilation strategy to reduce the risk of atelectasis and hypoxemia for obese patients undergoing surgery. Wang et al. [15] in a recent meta-analysis show that a strategy based on volume-controlled ventilation, positive end expiratory pressure (PEEP), and lung recruitment maneuvers was superior to other strategies in improving oxygenation, respiratory mechanics, and prevention of postoperative atelectasis in obese patients.

13.5 Postoperative Care Management

13.5.1 Postoperative Analgesia

The management of postoperative analgesia in OSA patients is a challenge for anesthetists. The use of major opioids (e.g., morphine, buprenorphine, and oxycodone) should be avoided or reduced, regardless of the method of administration. When the administration of morphine is indispensable, additive/synergic drugs must be used (e.g., ketamine, ketorolac) to reduce the dose in a multimodal analgesia strategy. The use of minor opioids is to be preferred to major analgesics. The administration of nonsteroidal anti-inflammatory drugs (NSAIDs) and paracetamol (acetaminophen) should be prescribed at regular times rather than "as needed." Use of patient-controlled analgesia (low-dose opioid continuous infusions when appropriate and necessary) depends on local protocols (infusion pumps versus elastomeric) and other logistical concerns. Our protocol provides the use of elastomeric infusion pumps with low-dose morphine and ketorolac for 48 h in patients with temporary tracheotomy. In all others we avoid major opioids using paracetamol at pre-established times with tramadol as rescue analgesic. We did not report adverse events related to analgesia in our experience.

In North America most patients are discharged home on postoperative day 1 or 2; they are given different combinations of narcotics (oxycodone elixir, dilaudid, hydrocodone) as well as topical analgesics (viscous lidocaine) and in some cases gabapentin, steroids, and COX 2 inhibitors. No one has an ideal way to manage postoperative pain.

13.5.2 Patient Bed Position

The importance of the patient's position in bed must not be underestimated. A 30° up-right position during the patient's stay in the recovery room (RR) and in the ward increases upper airway stability [16]. It is suggested that postoperative instructions should also specify the position to be maintained.

13.5.3 Oxygenation and CPAP

The authors agree on the need to administer oxygen to maintain preoperative saturation levels in patients who have previously received O_2 therapy. The administration of O_2 is not to be undertaken or must be interrupted when the patient, despite being confined to the bed, is able to maintain preoperative saturation levels in air environment. O_2 therapy should be administered continuously until the patient is able to maintain preoperative saturation values in air environment. It appears that the constant use of CPAP before and after surgical operation is the best strategy for the reduction of complications in the postoperative phase. However, CPAP is unable to guarantee patient safety in case of apnea caused by the administration of opioids. The use of noninvasive ventilation with backup respiratory frequency (e.g., assisted/controlled ventilation, pressure assist-control ventilation) may be advisable.

13.5.4 Ward or Intensive Care Unit?

Although OSA patients require adequate monitoring and surveillance, especially during the first 24 postoperative hours, there is a lack of evidence on the most appropriate duration of postoperative respiratory monitoring. Ideally the decision whether to admit patients to intensive care unit (ICU), or the ward, or to discharge them should be made before the surgical operation, although it can be made in the recovery room. These considerations should be correlated with the patient's need for analgesics as well as each institution's capability to monitor difficult airway patients (ICU, monitored intermediate care unit, monitored bed with expert nursing, ward, etc.) There is evidence to suggest that the occurrence of respiratory events in the RR foretells the recurrence of adverse events in the postoperative phase. Observation of recurring respiratory events in the RR may be used as an indicator to determine whether OSA or high-risk patients require continuous postoperative monitoring [17]. Figure 13.4 shows the algorithm of Italian Society of Anesthesia, Analgesia, Resuscitation and Intensive Care (SIAARTI)/Italian Association of Sleep Medicine (AIMS) Recommendations.

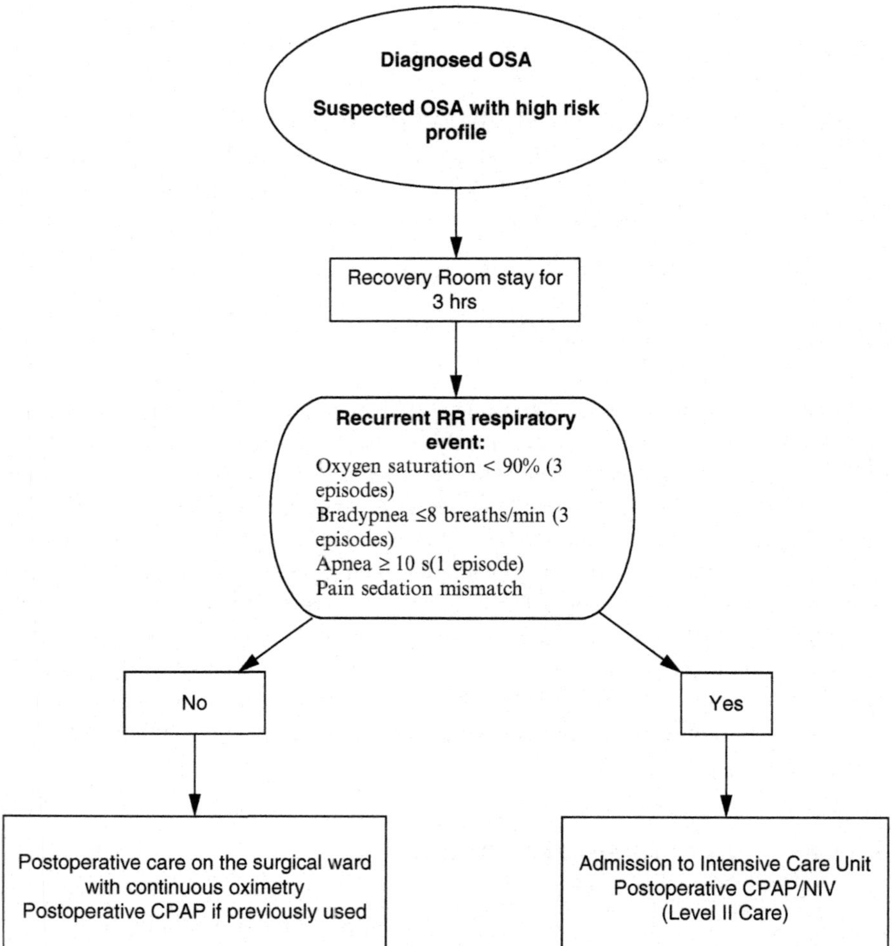

Fig. 13.4 The algorithm of Italian Society of Anesthesia, Analgesia, Resuscitation and Intensive Care (SIAARTI)/Italian Association of Sleep Medicine (AIMS) Recommendations

13.6 Special Topic: The Role of Tracheostomy

A temporary tracheostomy may be used to ensure airway patency after TORS, avoiding admission to the surgical ICU for mechanical ventilation and sedation to tolerate the endotracheal tube. In our experience a temporary tracheotomy is not always necessary, but for patients with severe OSAHS, severe comorbid conditions, BMI more than 30, and a narrow mouth opening, a planned tracheostomy is recommended for post-op ventilation assistance, especially if multi-level surgery has been performed. One more key reason for performing a planned tracheostomy is the degree of difficulty of re-intubation if the patient develops postsurgical airway edema or postoperative bleeding. Percutaneous dilation tracheostomy (PDT) has been compared extensively to surgical tracheostomy (ST), with a favorable profile characterized by fewer wound infections, lower rates of clinically significant bleeding, and significant cost savings [18]. This procedure entails bronchoscopic-guided insertion of a needle into the trachea, followed by insertion of a guidewire into the lumen, and then serial dilation via Seldinger technique. The final insertion is the tracheotomy tube (Fig. 13.5). Relative contraindications for PDT include, but are not limited to, coagulopathy, inability to extend the neck, c-spine instability, aberrant neck vasculature, distortion of the anterior tracheal anatomy, and overlying cellulitis. Although safe and effective, PDT is not without risk. Of complications known to be associated with PDT, trachea-innominate artery fistulas and posterior tracheal injury tend to be the most feared.

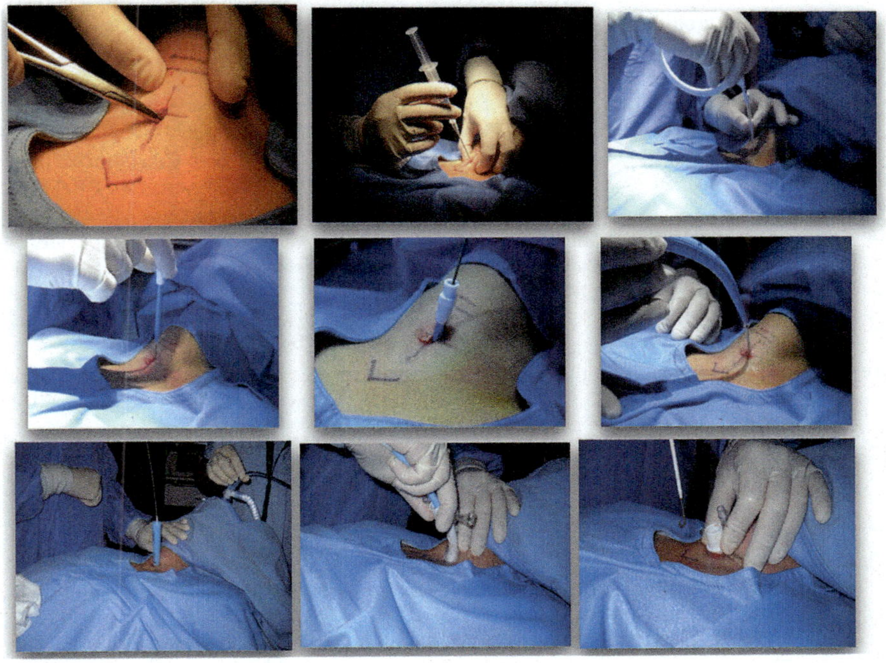

Fig. 13.5 Percutaneous tracheostomy performed in operating room

13.7 Conclusion

A patient affected by obstructive sleep apnea syndrome undergoing TORS is a patient at high risk from adverse events in the perioperative phase, which can be avoided only by the implementation of a well-defined clinical algorithm and a precise communication between anesthesiologist, surgeon, and nursing team.

References

1. Kaw R, Chung F, Pasupuleti V, Mehta J, Gay PC, Hernandez AV. Meta-analysis of the association between obstructive sleep apnoea and postoperative outcome. Br J Anaesth. 2012;109(6):897–906.
2. Ramachandran SK, Haider N, Saran KA, Mathis M, Kim J, Morris M, O'Reilly M. Life threatening critical respiratory events: a retrospective study of postoperative patients found unresponsive during analgesic therapy. J Clin Anesth. 2011;23(3):207–13.
3. American Society of Anesthesiologists Task Force on Perioperative Management of patients with obstructive sleep apnea. Practice guidelines for the perioperative management of patients with obstructive sleep apnea: an updated report by the American Society of Anesthesiologists Task Force on Perioperative Management of patients with obstructive sleep apnea. Anesthesiology. 2014;120(2):268–86.
4. Documento Intersocietario: Raccomandazioni SIAARTI-AIMS per la gestione perioperatoria del paziente affetto da Sindrome delle Apnee Ostruttive del Sonno. http://www.siaarti.it/corsi-patrocini/linee-guida-raccomandazioni/.
5. De Hert S, Imberger G, Carlisle J, Diemunsch P, Fritsch G, Moppett I, Solca M, Staender S, Wappler F, Smith A. Task Force on Preoperative Evaluation of the Adult Noncardiac Surgery Patient of the European Society of Anesthesiology. Preoperative evaluation of the adult patient undergoing non-cardiac surgery: guidelines from the European Society of Anesthesiology. Eur J Anesthesiol. 2011;28(10):684–722.
6. Corso RM, Petrini F, Buccioli M, et al. Clinical utility of preoperative screening with STOP-Bang questionnaire in elective surgery. Minerva Anestesiol. 2014;80(8):877–84.
7. Cattano D, Killoran PV, Cai C, Katsiampoura AD, Corso RM, Hagberg CA. Difficult mask ventilation in general surgical population: observation of risk factors and predictors. F1000Res. 2014;3:204.
8. Cattano D, Melnikov V, Khalil Y, Sridhar S, Hagberg CA. An evaluation of the rapid airway management positioner in obese patients undergoing gastric bypass or laparoscopic gastric banding surgery. Obes Surg. 2010;20(10):1436–41.
9. El-Ganzouri AR, McCarthy RJ, Tuman KJ, et al. Preoperative airway assessment: predictive value of a multivariate risk index. Anesth Analg. 1996;82:1197–204.
10. Corso RM, Cattano D, Buccioli M, Carretta E, Maitan S. Post analysis simulated correlation of the El Ganzouri Airway Difficulty score with difficult airway. Rev Bras Anestesiol. 2014. doi:10.1016/j.bjane.2014.09.003.
11. Cortellazzi P, Minati L, Falcone C, Lamperti M, Caldiroli D. Predictive value of the El-Ganzouri multivariate risk index for difficult tracheal intubation: a comparison of Glidescope videolaryngoscopy and conventional Macintosh laryngoscopy. Br J Anesth. 2007;99(6):906–11.
12. Cattano D, Corso RM, Altamirano AV, Patel CB, Meese MM, Seitan C, Hagberg CA. Clinical evaluation of the C-MAC D-Blade video laryngoscope in severely obese patients: a pilot study. Br J Anesth. 2012;109(4):647–8.
13. Popat M, Mitchell V, Dravid R, Patel A, Schampillai C, Higgs A. Difficult Airway Society Guidelines for the management of tracheal extubation. Anesthesia. 2012;67:318–40.

14. Ankichetty S, Wong J, Chung F. A systematic review of the effects of sedatives and anesthetics in patients with obstructive sleep apnea. J Anesthesiol Clin Pharmacol. 2011;27(4):447–58.
15. Wang C, Zhao N, Wang W, Guo L, Guo L, Chi C, Wang X, Pi X, Cui Y, Li E. Intraoperative mechanical ventilation strategies for obese patients: a systematic review and network meta-analysis. Obes Rev. 2015;16(6):508–17.
16. Neill AM, Angus SM, Sajkov D, McEvoy RD. Effects of sleep posture on upper airway stability in patients with obstructive sleep apnea. Am J Respir Crit Care Med. 1997;155:199–204.
17. Gali B, Whalen FX, Schroeder DR, Gay PC, Plevak DJ. Identification of patients at risk for postoperative respiratory complications using a preoperative obstructive sleep apnea screening tool and post-anesthesia care assessment. Anesthesiology. 2009;110(4):869–77.
18. Putensen C, Theuerkauf N, Guenther U, Vargas M, Pelosi P. Percutaneous and surgical tracheostomy in critically ill adult patients: a meta-analysis. Crit Care. 2014;18(6):544.

Chapter 14
Technique: How We Do It

Claudio Vicini, Filippo Montevecchi, and J. Scott Magnuson

14.1 Introduction

The unsurpassed visualisation, dexterity and control provided by the Da Vinci Surgical System® offer the following benefits for the surgeon: superior exposure and 3D HD visualisation of the target anatomy inside the pharynx, more precise dissection and improved preservation of intra-lingual vessels and nerves, shorter learning curve, faster operative time and a more reproducible approach as compared to traditional open as well as endoscopic techniques [1–5]. It also offers significant patient benefits: excellent cosmetic outcomes, no neck scars (except for tracheostomy, if necessary) [6, 7], reduced likelihood of iatrogenic injury to vessels and nerves, better and faster functional recovery compared to the trans-cervical approach, reduced operating room time and shortened length of hospital stay.

14.2 Exposure

The patient is positioned supine in the sniffing position (neck flexed and head extended) in order to achieve the best exposure. External compression manoeuvres can be used in order to enhance the exposure of different areas during the dissection (hyoid compression or other manoeuvres). Tongue base exposure is achieved in the standard

C. Vicini, M.D. • F. Montevecchi, M.D. (✉)
Head and Neck Department - ENT & Oral Surgery Unit - G.B. Morgagni - L. Pierantoni Hospital, Forlì – Infermi Hospital, Faenza - ASL of Romagna, Italy
e-mail: claudio@claudiovicini.com; filippomontevecchi72@gmail.com; filo651@hotmail.com

J.S. Magnuson, M.D.
Head and Neck Surgery Department, Florida Hospital Celebration Health, Celebration, FL, USA
e-mail: scott.magnuson.md@flhosp.org

© Springer International Publishing Switzerland 2016

C. Vicini et al. (eds.), *TransOral Robotic Surgery for Obstructive Sleep Apnea*, DOI 10.1007/978-3-319-34040-1_14

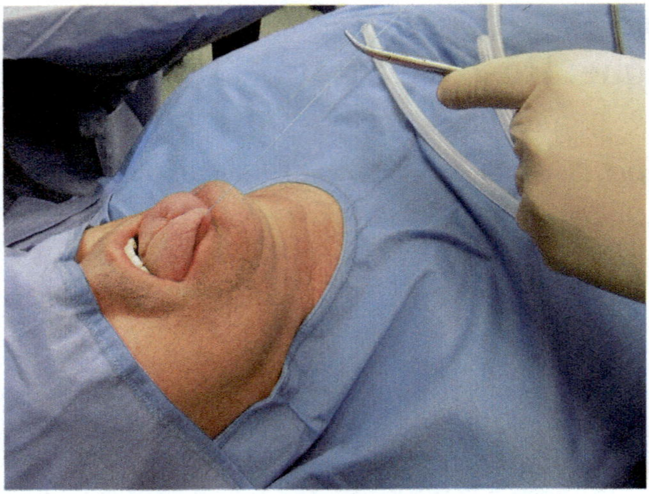

Fig. 14.1 Tongue base exposure is achieved in the standard TORS approach with a combination of tongue tip traction (0 silk stitch horizontal mattress suture) and tongue body displacement by mouth gag

TORS approach with a combination of tongue tip traction (with a 0 silk stitch horizontal mattress suture) (Fig. 14.1) and tongue body displacement by Storz, Davis Meyer® mouth gag under direct visualisation with a head light. A complete set of tongue blades of different sizes with integrated suction tubes (for smoke and blood) is of paramount importance (Fig. 14.2). A small, wide blade has proven to be the most suitable tool in most cases (Storz blade number 1 and 2). In patients with significant macroglossia the smaller and narrower blade may cause significant lateral in-rolling of the tongue body margins. In this situation the working space will be reduced and the introduction of the robotic arms may be difficult. The use of a longer and wider blade (Storz blade number 3) is possible in order to prevent lateral tongue body prolapse into the surgical field. In cases of macroglossia the tongue is partially released in order to allow adequate exposure of the tongue base. A combination of tongue base traction and properly selected mouth gag blade length is the key for excellent exposure. Repositioning of the tongue blade during the resection is rarely necessary. However, it may be helpful to remove and reposition the tongue blade after the resection is complete; this strategy will ensure that lingual tonsil tissue is not inadvertently missed resulting in inadequate resection. Usually the short or the medium blade (Storz blade number 1 and 2) is very effective for completing tongue base as well as epiglottis procedures. If a second blade is to be inserted after the initial resection, the new position must be carefully verified in order to avoid the loss of proper orientation. The 12 mm 30° 3D scope (upward facing) is our preferred choice. If available an 8 mm scope may be very helpful in particular cases (minimal inter-incisive distance, extreme macroglossia, etc.). Only two robotic 5 mm Endo Wrist® are routinely used for each patient: a Maryland Dissector for grasping and dissecting tissues and a monopolar cautery with a spatula tip for dissection and coagulation.

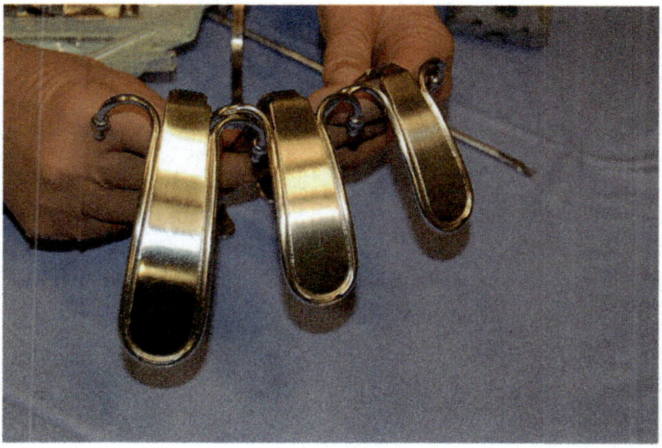

Fig. 14.2 Complete set of tongue blades of different sizes with integrated suction tubes (for smoke and blood)

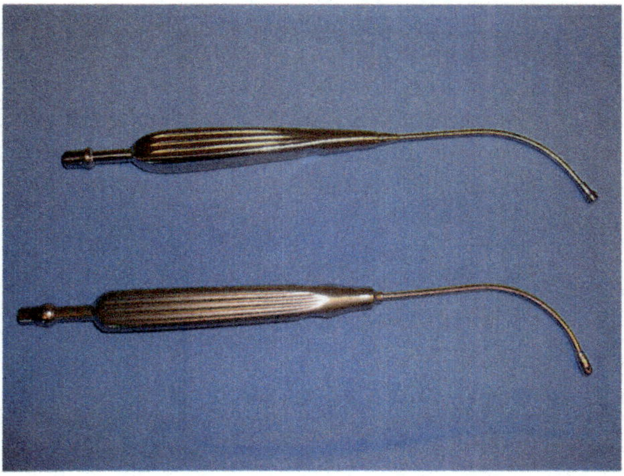

Fig. 14.3 Bedside assistant's suction devices (Lawton suction® Cat. 160274 and/or Medicon suction® Cat. 098508), which can be used for retraction and the evacuation of smoke and blood

Surgical clip placement is usually not required, but in special cases clipping of large vessels may prove to be very helpful. Additional hemostasis can be provided by using an insulated coagulation-suction tube (Storz® Cat. 12067R). An insulated bipolar forceps (Storz® Cat. 842219) is of paramount importance for safe coagulation in the peripheral aspects of the surgical field. The forceps must be insulated from the tip to the handle in order to avoid burns of the oral commissure. A Neurosurgical Malis Bipolar® (Codman) or a bipolar Dessi® (Microfrance) coagulating device originally studied for sinus surgery may be helpful as well. The bedside assistant provides two additional suction devices (Lawton suction® Cat. 160274 and/or Medicon suction® Cat. 098508) (Fig. 14.3), which can be used for retraction and the evacuation of smoke and blood.

14.3 Surgical Steps

TORS approach for OSA may include three different surgical steps frequently combined in the same procedures according to the patient's features [8–10]. These steps will be described in detail:

Tongue base reduction (TBR)
Supraglottoplasty (SGP)
Anterior midline glossectomy (AMG)

14.3.1 Tongue Base Reduction

The goal of TBR is to enlarge the oropharyngeal space by removing tissue from the anterior wall. The end point of TBR may be achieved when the surgical view changes from a Cormack & Lehane Grade IV or III to a Grade II or I [11, 12]. In most cases lymphoid tissue as well as tongue base muscle must be removed in order to clear the retro-lingual space or posterior airway space (PAS). In case of massive lymphoid hyperplasia less muscular tissue needs to be removed. Conversely, if the lingual tonsils are not enlarged then a more aggressive muscular resection is required in order to obtain the Cormack & Lehane Grade II/I. The mean volume of tissue removed is typically 10 ml, but in some cases the overall volume may be up to 50 ml. The surgical steps are standardised in a precise and logical sequence, and are described in detail.

14.3.1.1 Right-Side Lingual Tonsillectomy

Instrument setting:	**Maryland left**
	Monopolar right
	Setting: coagulation/blended (no cutting)
	Energy level (15–30) according to the device

The procedure starts with a midline split of the two lingual tonsils from foramen caecum in order to identify the tip of epiglottis and vallecula (Fig. 14.4). The dissection is carried out using monopolar cautery until the junction between lymphatic tissue and muscle is identified. In patients with extreme lingual tonsil hypertrophy it may be difficult to identify the foramen caecum and circumvallate papilla. In these cases debulking of the midline lymphoid tissue may help the surgeon to identify the essential surgical landmarks. At the beginning of the dissection it is strongly recommended that the surgeon position the tip of the scope far from the tongue base in order to provide a wide surgical view under low magnification; this will enhance the surgeon's 3D

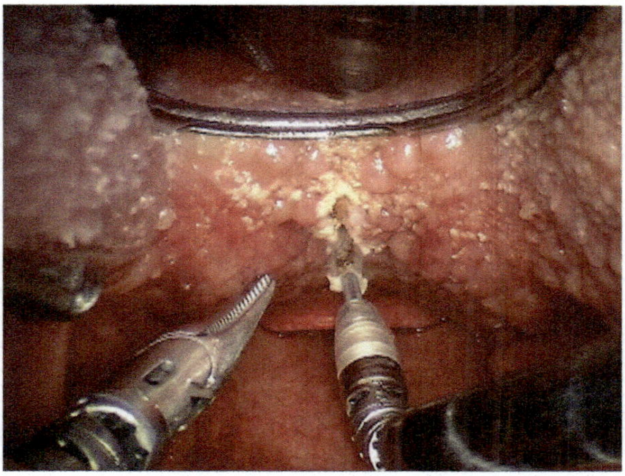

Fig. 14.4 The procedure starts with a midline split of the two lingual tonsils from foramen caecum in order to identify the tip of epiglottis and vallecular

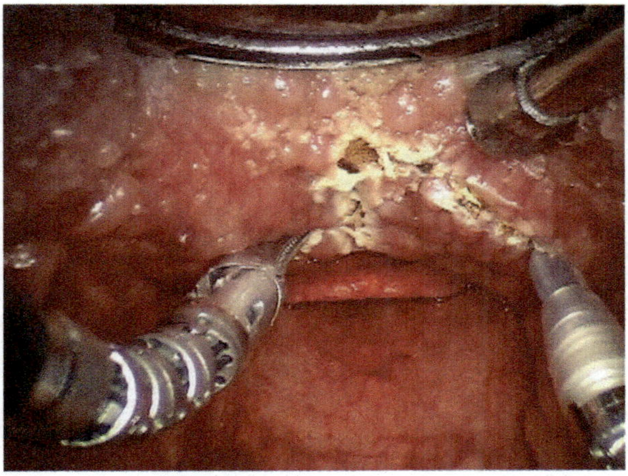

Fig. 14.5 Initial dissection of the right tongue base posteriorly to the circumvallate papilla

awareness of the anatomy (Fig. 14.5). At the end of this first step, the lingual tonsils are completely divided in the midline creating a deep groove joining the foramen caecum superiorly to the glosso-epiglottic ligament inferiorly. Dissection is carried out using the tip of the spatula, "painting" layer by layer through the tissue in order to maintain direct visualization of the tip of the instrument. In order to grasp the tissue a deep cut must be created to allow the Maryland forceps to gain adequate purchase of the tissue; otherwise repeated attempts of grasping will produce tedious, excessive bleeding (Fig. 14.6). In cases of mild to moderate lingual tonsil hyperplasia, after midline dissection, the superior (sulcus terminalis), lateral (glosso-tonsillar sulcus), and inferior (glosso-epiglottic sulcus) borders of the right lingual tonsil are identified and marked by cautery. In cases of extreme lingual tonsil hyperplasia, after midline splitting, it is recommended to perform a midline lingual tonsil debulking in order to allow better manipulation and better identification of the limit of the dissection. If lingual tonsil hyperplasia is mild to moderate, the right lingual tonsillectomy is

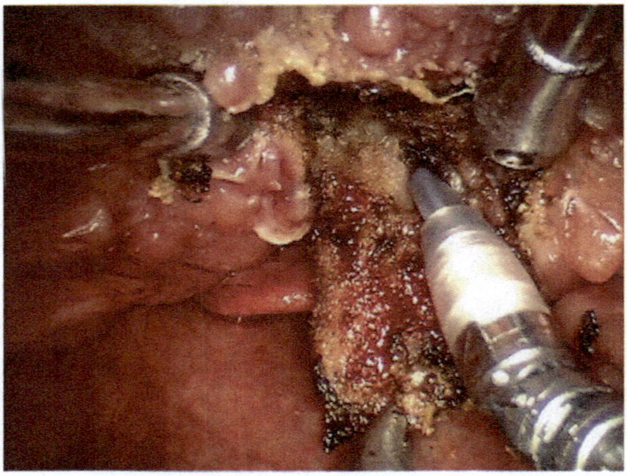

Fig. 14.6 In order to grasp the tissue a deep cut must be created to allow the Maryland forceps to gain adequate purchase of the tissue

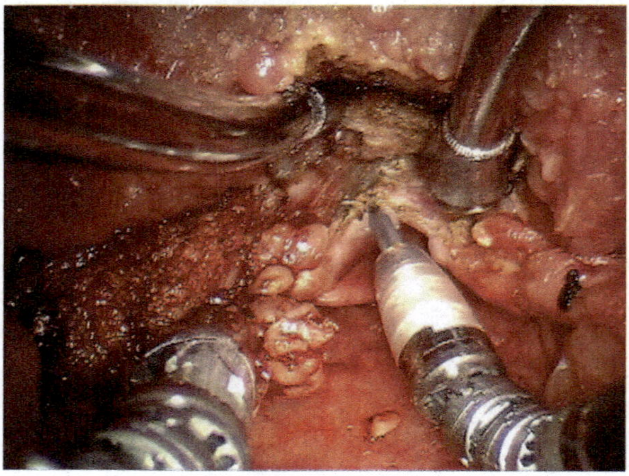

Fig. 14.7 Bedside assistant maintains counter-traction in order to assist the surgeon during dissection; increased tension allows more precise and quicker dissection

performed "en bloc" superiorly to inferiorly maintaining the dissection plane close to the lympho-muscular junction. During this step the scope is positioned closer to the surgical field for better identification of neurovascular structures. Bleeding during these phase of the dissection is usually minimal. Additional remarks:

- A precise multidimensional resection is easily performed with the 3D view of the da Vinci optics.
- Bedside assistant maintains counter-traction in order to assist the surgeon during dissection; increased tension allows more precise and quicker dissection (Fig. 14.7).
- The inferior limit of the resection is characterised by a bluish colour representing the vallecular mucosa and by an increased bleeding.

14.3.1.2 Left-Sided Lingual Tonsillectomy

Instrument setting:	Maryland right
	Monopolar left
	Setting: coagulation/blended (no cutting)
	Energy level (15–30) according to the device

After completing right lingual tonsillectomy (Fig. 14.8) left lingual tonsillectomy is completed in the same way after side inversion of the robotic tools (Figs. 14.9 and 14.10).

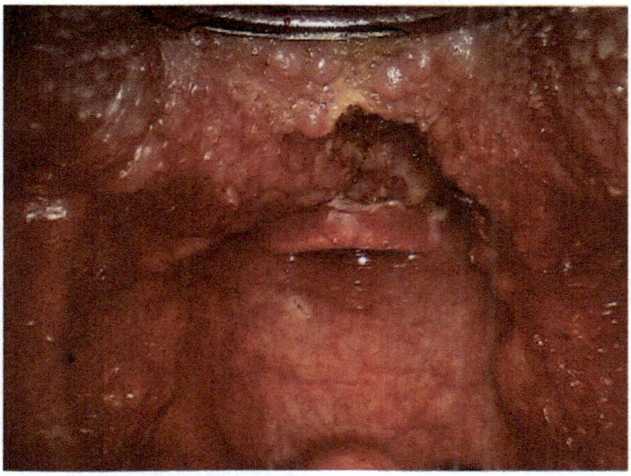

Fig. 14.8 Surgical field after right lingual tonsillectomy

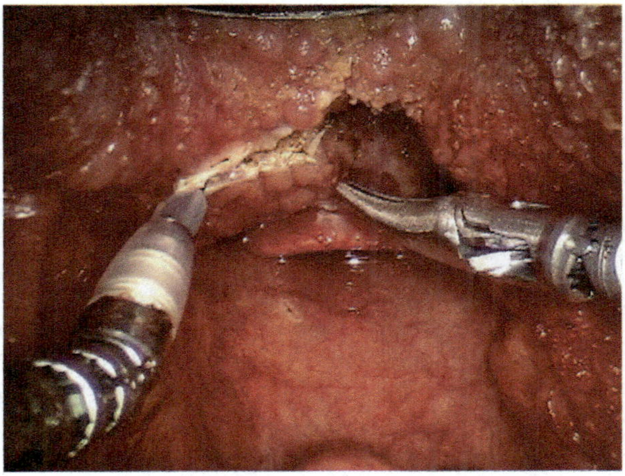

Fig. 14.9 Left lingual tonsillectomy is completed in the same way of the right after side inversion of the robotic arms and tools. Initial mucosa dissection

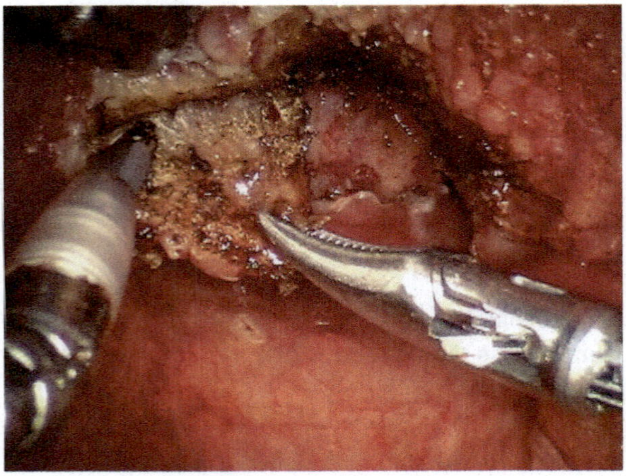

Fig. 14.10 Left lingual tonsillectomy is completed in the same way of the right after side inversion of the robotic arms and tools. Dissection of deeper layers

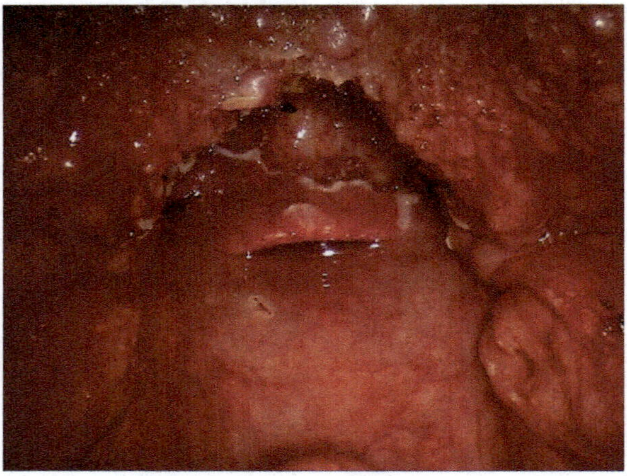

Fig. 14.11 Surgical field at the end of the lingual tonsillectomy. At this step a view of the epiglottis is possible

14.3.1.3 Residual Obstruction Evaluation

The surgical field is now inspected in order to evaluate the residual degree of obstruction (Fig. 14.11). If Cormack & Lehane Grade is greater than 2, additional resection in the muscle layer is required. Additional information is provided by the volume of tissue resected and measured using a graduated syringe filled with saline. If the overall volume of resected tissue is less than 7 ml an additional resection may be recommended. Repositioning of the tongue blade or replacement of the tongue blade with a larger and or smaller blade may assist the surgeon by exposing tissue that may have been compressed by the retractor.

14.3.1.4 Additional Resections

In order to open the posterior airway space it may be necessary to remove muscle in addition to lymphoid tissue. When entering the muscular layer it is important to avoid injury to the neurovascular structures including the dorsal branches of the lingual arteries and hypoglossal nerve. A number of investigators have published interesting cadaveric dissections [10, 13–15] describing practical anatomical landmarks in this area. Woodson stresses the importance of intraoperative mapping of the tongue vasculature using ultrasound if available. Most authors would agree that anatomical landmarks are unreliable due to great individual anatomic variability and to the extreme mobility of the active tongue. In addition the tongue shape is modified in the surgical setting due to retraction and positioning [16]. In our experience two additional points must be stressed:

- The relationship of the lingual artery and hyoid bone is a reliable landmark and is described in the surgical anatomy chapter.
- The 3D HD da Vinci® camera allows for the identification of the crucial structures before damaging them, *working carefully step by step, with a mix of blunt and sharp dissection* (Figs. 14.12 and 14.13).

The overall time required for TBR is about 30 min.

14.3.2 Supraglottoplasty

SGP may be carried out concurrently with TBR in patients with primary and in some cases secondary epiglottic collapse. The role of SGP is to prevent the inward collapse of the floppy epiglottis and/or redundant supraglottic tissue. The additional time required for SPG is usually less than 15 min. The most common procedure in supraglottic area includes the following steps:

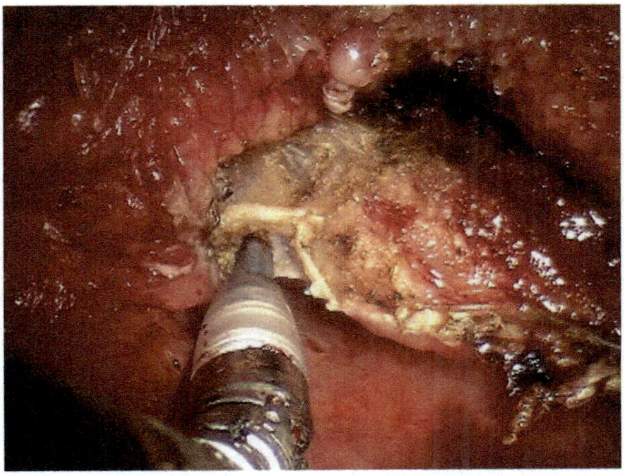

Fig. 14.12 In case of additional resection of muscle the 3D HD da Vinci® camera allows for the identification of the crucial structures before damaging them, working carefully step by step, with a mix of blunt and sharp dissection

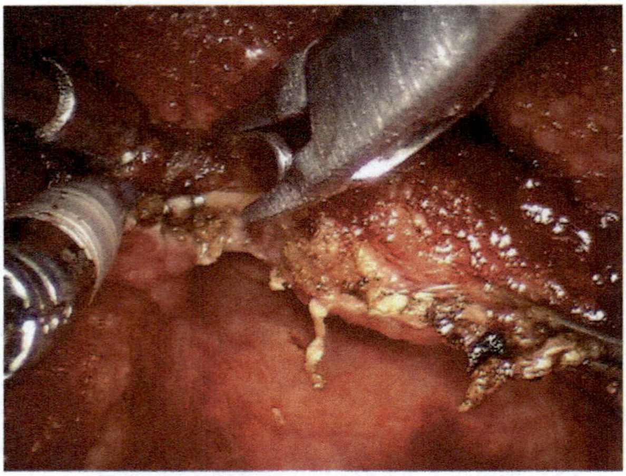

Fig. 14.13 A vessel clip applier or an insulated bipolar forceps used by the bedside assistant can manage intra-operative bleeding

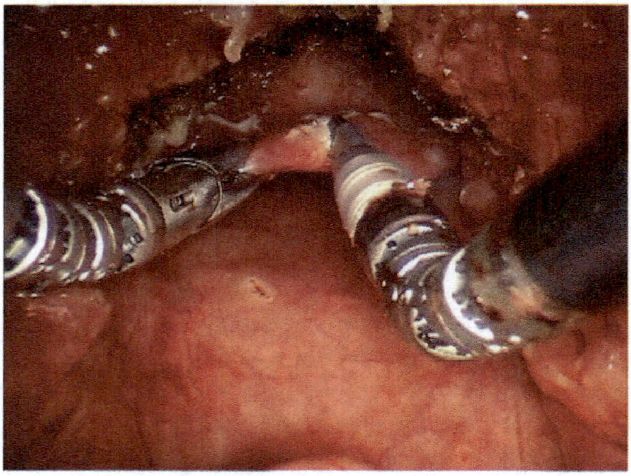

Fig. 14.14 Vertical midline splitting of supra-hyoid epiglottis

- *Vertical midline splitting of supra-hyoid epiglottis (Fig. 14.14)*: This step is carried out along the midline, following the medial glosso-epiglottic fold, from the tip of the epiglottis inferiorly, preserving at least 5 mm of epiglottis above the deep vallecular plane (a sufficient remnant of epiglottic cartilage is left to avoid aspiration).
- *A horizontal section is performed bilaterally* in a plane joining the vertical section in the midline and running laterally immediately over the pharyngo-epiglottic fold, in order to leave a lateral fold preventing aspiration, and in order to avoid possible bleeding from the superior laryngeal vessels (Figs. 14.15, 14.16, 14.17, and 14.18): Scarring of the vallecular and peri-vallecular area leads to progressive adhesion and stabilisation of the residual epiglottis to the tongue base.
- A modification of the previously described procedure as described by Magnuson (unpublished data) is the *"V-shape" epiglottoplasty*. A V-shape wedge is removed from the central epiglottis. This technique is probably safer for the airway and for the superior laryngeal vascular bundle.

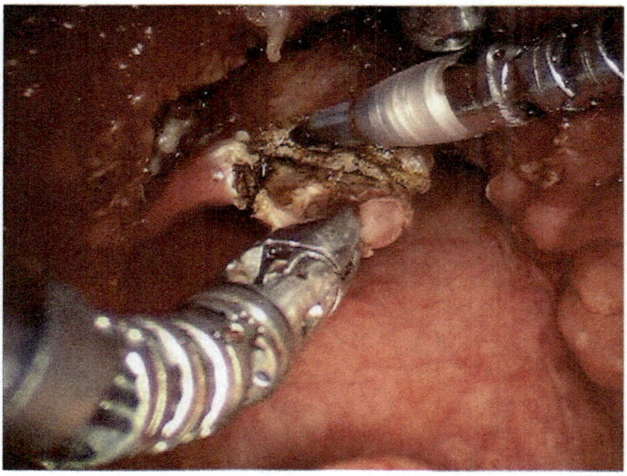

Fig. 14.15 Right lateral dissection of the epiglottis immediately over the pharyngo-epiglottic fold

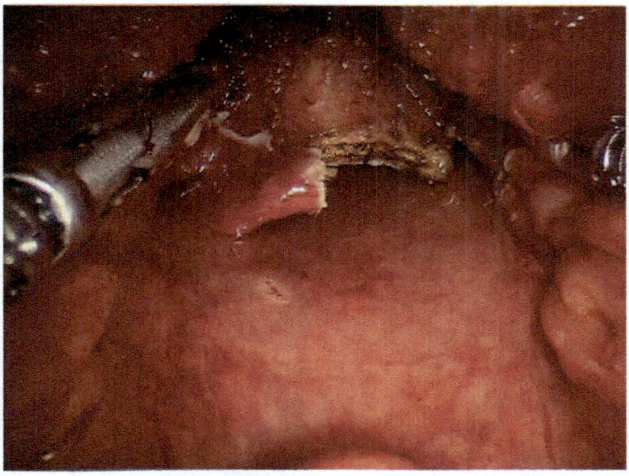

Fig. 14.16 Surgical field at the end of the right epiglottoplasty

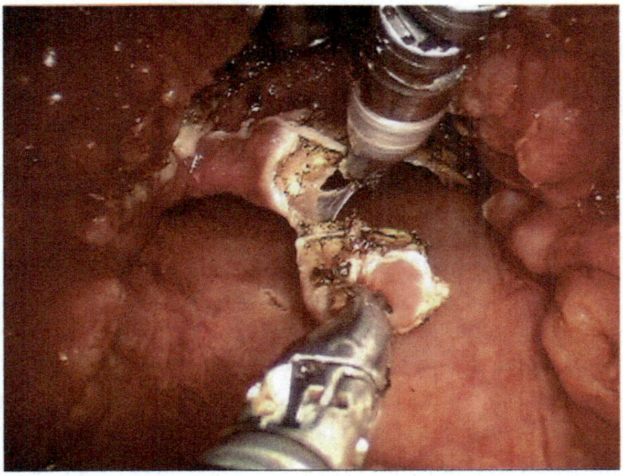

Fig. 14.17 Left lateral dissection of the epiglottis immediately over the pharyngo-epiglottic fold

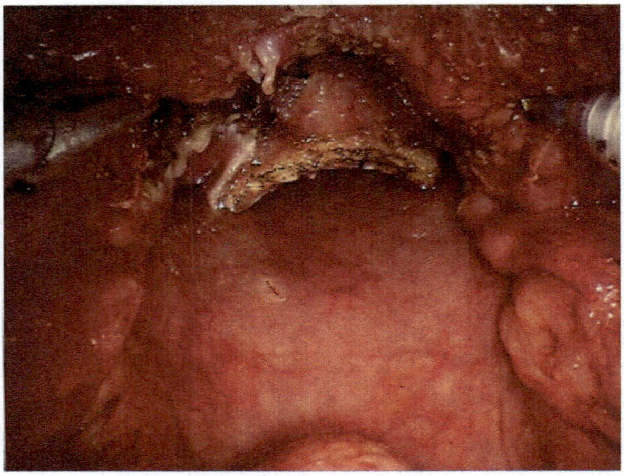

Fig. 14.18 Surgical field at the end of the epiglottoplasty

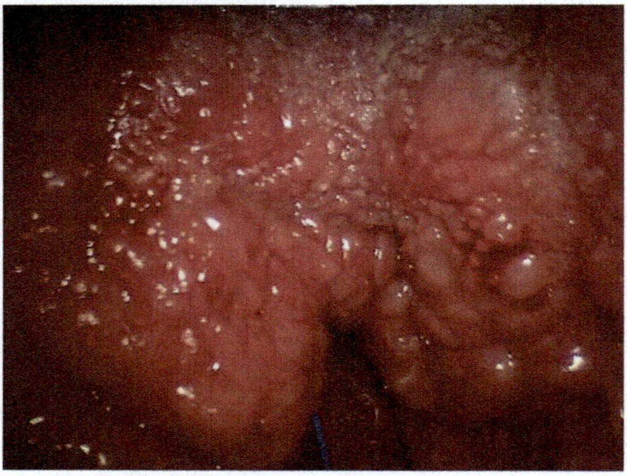

Fig. 14.19 Tongue base reduction and supraglottoplasty in patient with nasotracheal intubation and extreme lingual tonsil hypertrophy

The surgical steps shown in Figs. 14.19, 14.20, 14.21, 14.22, 14.23, and 14.24 have been performed in patients who haven't undergone planned preoperative tracheostomy. Tracheostomy is not performed routinely for patients undergoing TORS, but is performed in certain circumstances: (1) patients who were found to have a difficult intubation, and (2) situations where emergent reintubation is anticipated to be difficult. It is important to understand that tracheostomy is not performed solely due to an enlarged tongue base. In most cases, surgeon preference dictates either trans-nasal or trans-oral intubation for benign base of tongue TORS procedures. Consultation with the anesthesia provider about the possibility of tracheostomy should be discussed both before and after intubation. Although unplanned tracheostomy is rare, patients should be aware and consented for this possibility.

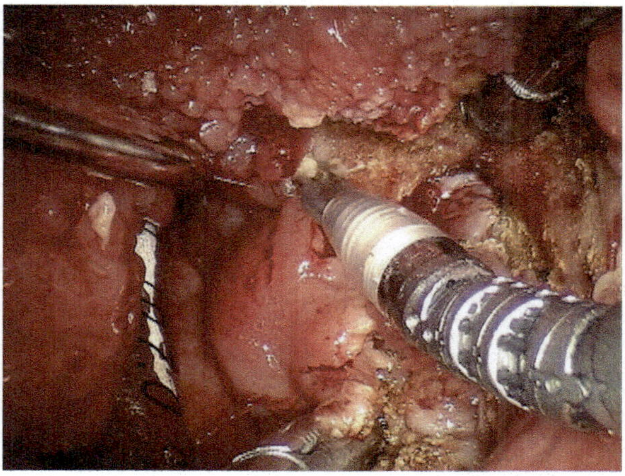

Fig. 14.20 Dissection of the right tongue base

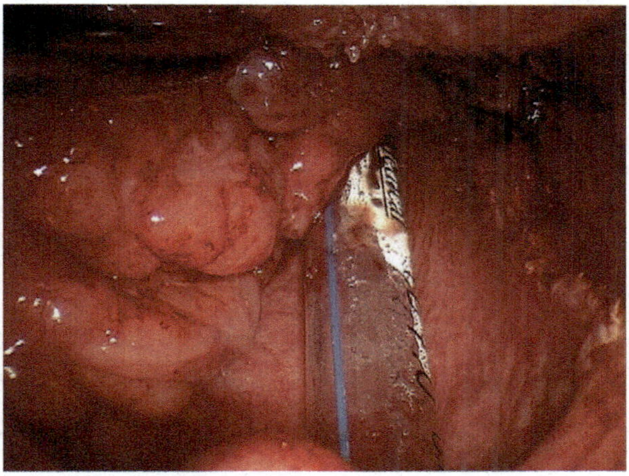

Fig. 14.21 Surgical field at the end of the right tongue base reduction

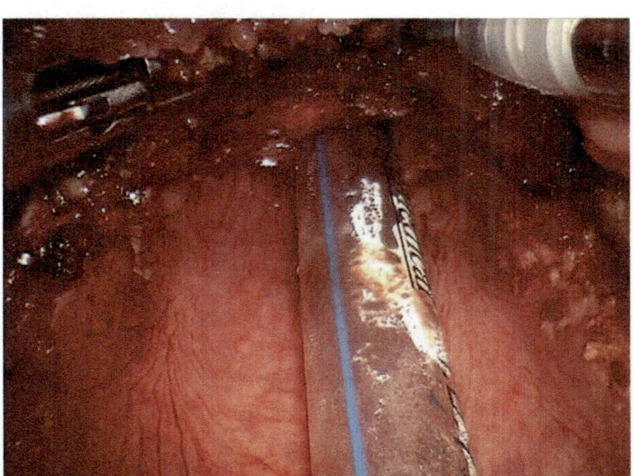

Fig. 14.22 Surgical field at the end of the tongue base reduction

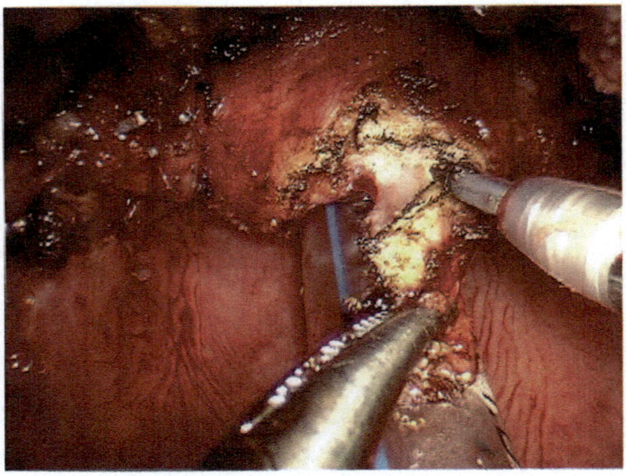

Fig. 14.23 Right lateral dissection of the epiglottis

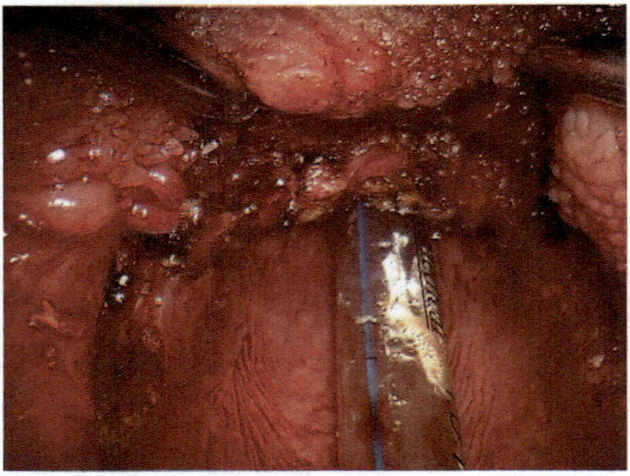

Fig. 14.24 Surgical field at the end of the epiglottoplasty

14.3.3 Anterior Midline Glossectomy

In selected cases of oral tongue macroglossia an extended anterior resection is possible in the midline area anterior to the circumvallate papilla. This additional removal of muscle tissue usually requires the sacrifice of the central circumvallate papillae, with minimal functional impact, and is carried out between the branches of the lingual artery. At the completion of the midline dissection, the wound is closed using absorbable suture. A special set of customised tongue blades provides optimal exposure of the midline area (not yet commercially available).

References

1. Chabolle F, Wagner I, Blumen MB, et al. Tongue base reduction with hyoepigottoplasty: a treatment for severe obstructive sleep apnea. Laryngoscope. 1999;109(8):1273–80.
2. Blumen MB, Coquille F, Rocchicioli C, Mellot F, Chabolle F. Radiofrequency tongue reduction through a cervical approach: a pilot study. Laryngoscope. 2006;116(10):1887–93.
3. Friedman M, Soans R, Gurpinar B, Lin HC, Joseph N. Evaluation of submucosal minimally invasive lingual excision technique for treatment of obstructive sleep apnea/hypopnea syndrome. Otolaryngol Head Neck Surg. 2008;139(3):378–84.
4. Fujita S, Woodson BT, Clark JL, Wittig R. Laser midline glossectomy as a treatment for obstructive sleep apnea. Laryngoscope. 1991;101(8):805–9.
5. Mickelson S, Rosenthal L. Midline glossectomy and epiglottidectomy for obstructive sleep apnea syndrome. Laryngoscope. 1997;107(5):614–9.
6. Campanini A, De Vito A, Frassineti S, Vicini C. Temporary tracheotomy in the surgical treatment of obstructive sleep apnea syndrome: personal experience. Acta Otorhinolaryngol Ital. 2003;23(6):474–8.
7. Sun H, Lou W, Wang L, Wu Y. Clinical significance of preoperative tracheotomy in preventing perioperative OSAHS severe complications. Lin Chuang Er Bi Yan Hou Ke Za Zhi. 2005;19(9):394–5.
8. Vicini C, Dallan I, Canzi P, Frassineti S, La Pietra MG, Montevecchi F. Transoral robotic tongue base resection in obstructive sleep apnoea-hypopnoea syndrome: a preliminary report. ORL J Otorhinolaryngol Relat Spec. 2010;72(1):22–7.
9. Vicini C, Montevecchi F, Tenti G, Canzi P, Dallan I, Huntley TC. Transoral robotic surgery: tongue base reduction and supraglottoplasty for obstructive sleep apnea. Oper Tech Otolaryngol Head Neck Surg. 2012;23(1):45–7.
10. Vicini C, Dallan I, Canzi P, et al. Transoral robotic surgery of the tongue base in obstructive sleep Apnea-Hypopnea syndrome: anatomic considerations and clinical experience. Head Neck. 2012;34:15–22.
11. Cormack RS, Lehane J. Difficult tracheal intubation in obstetrics. Anaesthesia. 1984;39(11):1105–11.
12. Yentis SM, Lee DJ. Evaluation of an improved scoring system for the grading of direct laryngoscopy. Anaesthesia. 1998;53(11):1041–4.
13. Sequert C, Lestang P, Baglin AC, Wagner I, Ferron JM, Chabolle F. Hypoglossal nerve in its intralingual trajectory: anatomy and clinical implications. Ann Otolaryngol Chir Cervicofac. 1999;116(4):207–17.
14. Lauretano AM, Li KK, Caradonna DS, Khosta RK, Fried MP. Anatomic location of the tongue base neurovascular bundle. Laryngoscope. 1997;107(8):1057–9.
15. O'Malley Jr BW, Weinstein GS, Snyder W, Hockstein NG. Transoral robotic surgery (TORS) for base of tongue neoplasms. Laryngoscope. 2006;116(8):1465–72.
16. Wu D, Qin J, Guo X, Li S. Analysis of the difference in the course of the lingual arteries caused by tongue position change. Laryngoscope. 2015;125(3):762–6.

Part III
Post-Operative Concerns

Chapter 15
Postoperative Management of Transoral Robotic Surgery for Obstructive Sleep Apnea

Chiara Marchi and Julia A. Crawford

15.1 Introduction

Obstructive sleep apnea (OSA) is the most common cause of sleep-disordered breathing with an increasing prevalence worldwide [1]. The incidence of perioperative complications is well known to be greater in patients with OSA than in the baseline population. This has led to the American Society of Anesthesiologists and the American Academy of Sleep Medicine developing clinical practice guidelines for the perioperative management of patients with OSA [2]. Patients who have had surgical intervention for their OSA are at even greater risk of perioperative events and understanding the potential impact of OSA on patients' surgical risk profile is of upmost importance. Post OSA surgery patients will have not only more difficult airway management but also have altered drug sensitivity, a higher risk of undiagnosed comorbid disease and the potential for operative site bleeding complicating an already difficult airway [3, 4].

C. Marchi, M.D. (✉)
Head and Neck Department—ENT & Oral Surgery Unit, G.B. Morgagni—L. Pierantoni Hospital, ASL of Romagna, Forlì, Italy

Infermi Hospital, ASL of Romagna, Faenza, Italy
e-mail: marchi.chiara@alice.it

J.A. Crawford, B.Sc., M.B.B.S., F.R.A.C.S.
Department of Otolaryngology, Head and Neck Surgery, St Vincent's Hospital, Darlinghurst, NSW, Australia
e-mail: drjuliacrawford@gmail.com

© Springer International Publishing Switzerland 2016

C. Vicini et al. (eds.), *TransOral Robotic Surgery for Obstructive Sleep Apnea*,
DOI 10.1007/978-3-319-34040-1_15

15.2 Perioperative Airway Management

OSA surgical patients, regardless of the surgical intervention undertaken are at increased risk of airway compromise secondary to instrumentation of the airway and increased risk of bleeding. Furthermore, anesthetic and sedative drugs are central nervous system depressants and additionally depress skeletal muscle tone increasing the tendency of the upper airway to collapse and worsening the severity of OSA [5]. All post upper airway surgical patients should be closely monitored regarding the risk of upper airway swelling and airway compromise.

During transoral robotic surgical (TORS) operations for OSA in Europe the airway has customarily been secured intraoperatively with a tracheostomy [6]. This is not routinely advocated in the US or Singapore, and surgery is more commonly performed via orotracheal or nasotracheal intubation [7]. Institutional guidelines from the Forlì University group in Italy stipulate that a temporary perioperative tracheostomy is required for all patients with severe OSA or in those patients who are undergoing multilevel surgical intervention regardless of OSA severity [8]. If the patient has not undergone tracheostomy placement, the patient is assessed for extubation at the end of the procedure. Overnight ICU stay with continued intubation followed by extubation in the operating room may be necessary depending on surgeon preference.

One risk specific to TORS is the risk of lingual swelling secondary to retractor placement. This swelling typically reaches its peak about 12–24 h after the operation. The degree of swelling seems to be related to the time spent in suspension. Limiting the time in suspension to less than one hour reduces this risk.

15.3 Acuity of Care

All patients operated on for OSA with TORS should be monitored closely in the early postoperative period for both the potential risk of bleeding and for the risk of airway edema. The patient should be monitored in an intensive or high-dependency care unit. Hypoxemia, hypercapnia, and hypertension are also important concerns in the postoperative period. As hypoxia is the main drive to producing arousal during apneic events, supplemental oxygen should be avoided [9]. Patients should have continuous oximetry monitoring, ECG, and blood pressure monitoring in the immediate postoperative. Typically, adverse airway related events will occur within the first 24 h after surgery. Patients may be downgraded to a lower acuity care day one postoperatively [10].

15.4 Pain and Nausea Management

Strategies for postoperative analgesia should emphasize the use of multimodality analgesic therapy. Anecdotal evidence implicates opioids as a risk factor for cardiorespiratory arrest in patients with severe OSA and should be used with caution

[11, 12]. However, this risk must be balanced against the needs of the patient. There are several analgesic adjuncts that can be used with opioid sparing properties such as tramadol, regular acetaminophen, dexmedetomidine, and pergabalin; the last two having both analgesic and anxiolytic properties [13]. Postoperative intravenous steroids can help with nausea, airway edema, and pain from the inflammatory response. It is advisable to continue oral steroids post-discharge on a tapering dose, as most patients experience a significant crescendo of pain up to a week postoperatively, likely due to hyperinflammation or dissolution of the fibrinous exudative protective coating over the surgical site. Antiemetic and antitussive drugs can be added to this treatment regime.

15.5 Dietary Management

Consideration should be given to placement of a nasogastric feeding tube, and some centers routinely use NG tubes for all TORS patients in the immediate postoperative period. The Forli University group have found that many patients can swallow liquids comfortably without aspiration within 1 day of surgery, but this can vary considerably between patients. The protocol in Forli is to commence a liquid diet supplemented with IV fluids postoperative day 1 then upgrading to more advanced diets depending on patient tolerance. The group have found that adequate swallowing is typically seen on average by 2.5 days after surgery. The need for a postoperative gastrostomy tube is rare and is correlated with those patients undergoing multiple concurrent procedures [14].

15.6 Conclusion

The postoperative management of TORS OSA patients is similar to those undergoing non-robotic upper airway surgery. It is important to remain cognizant that OSA patients undergoing any type of surgery are at increased risk of perioperative complications and those who have had upper airway surgery are at even greater risk. However, with appropriate postoperative care these risks can be minimized.

References

1. Peppard PE, Young T, Barnet JH, Palta M, Hagen EW, Hla KM. Increased prevalence of sleep-disordered breathing in adults. Am J Epidemiol. 2013;177(9):1006–14.
2. Practice guidelines for the perioperative management of patients with obstructive sleep apnea: an updated report by the American Society of Anesthesiologists Task Force on Perioperative Management of patients with obstructive sleep apnea. American Society of Anesthesiologists Task Force on Perioperative Management of patients with obstructive sleep apnea. Anesthesiology. 2014 Feb;120(2):268–86. doi:10.1097/ALN.0000000000000053.

3. Pedrosa RP, Drager LF, Gonzaga CC, Sousa MG, de Paula LKG, Amaro ACS, et al. Obstructive sleep apnea: the most common secondary cause of hypertension associated with resistant hypertension. Hypertension. 2011;58(5):811–7.
4. Resnick HE, Redline S, Shahar E, Gilpin A, Newman A, Walter R, et al. Diabetes and sleep disturbances: findings from the Sleep Heart Health Study. Diabetes Care. 2003;26(3):702–9.
5. Perioperative treatment of patients with obstructive sleep apnea. 2015 Oct 11;:1–7.
6. Vicini C, Dallan I, Canzi P, Frassineti S, Nacci A, Seccia V, et al. Transoral robotic surgery of the tongue base in obstructive sleep Apnea-Hypopnea syndrome: anatomic considerations and clinical experience. Head Neck. 2011;34(1):15–22.
7. White HN, Frederick J, Zimmerman T, Carroll WR, Magnuson JS. Learning curve for transoral robotic surgery: a 4-year analysis. JAMA Otolaryngol Head Neck Surg. 2013;139(6):564–7.
8. Vicini C, Montevecchi F, Tenti G, Canzi P, Dallan I, Huntley TC. Transoral robotic surgery: tongue base reduction and supraglottoplasty for obstructive sleep apnea. Oper Tech Otolaryngol Head Neck Surg. 2012;23(1):45–7.
9. Jain SS, Dhand R. Perioperative treatment of patients with obstructive sleep apnea. Curr Opin Pulm Med. 2004;10(6):482–8.
10. Hoff PT, D'Agostino MA, Thaler ER. Transoral robotic surgery in benign diseases including obstructive sleep apnea: safety and feasibility. Laryngoscope. 2015;125(5):1249–53.
11. Ostermeier AM, Roizen MF, Hautkappe M, Klock PA, Klafta JM. Three sudden postoperative respiratory arrests associated with epidural opioids in patients with sleep apnea. Anesth Analg. 1997;85(2):452–60.
12. Reeder MK, Goldman MD, Loh L, Muir AD, Casey KR, Gitlin DA. Postoperative obstructive sleep apnoea. Haemodynamic effects of treatment with nasal CPAP. Anaesthesia. 1991;46(10):849–53.
13. Brenner MJ, Goldman JL. Obstructive sleep apnea and surgery: quality improvement imperatives and opportunities. Curr Otorhinolaryngol Rep. 2014;2(1):20–9.
14. Glazer TA, Hoff PT, Spector ME. Transoral robotic surgery for obstructive sleep apnea. JAMA Otolaryngol Head Neck Surg. 2014;140(12):1207–6.

Chapter 16
Expected Outcomes

Claudio Vicini, Filippo Montevecchi, Aldo Campanini, Iacopo Dallan, Paul T. Hoff, Matthew E. Spector, Erica R. Thaler, Jeffrey Ahn, Peter M. Baptista, Marc Remacle, Georges Lawson, Marco Benazzo, and Pietro Canzi

16.1 Introduction

Transoral robotic surgery (TORS) for obstructive sleep apnea/hypopnea syndrome (OSAHS) was first performed in 2008 and published within a case series of patients [1]. While this report only included the preliminary experience in ten patients, it demonstrated feasibility and set the stage for expansion of this technology as well as the refinement of the technique. As of late 2014, it was estimated that more than 450 TORS cases were performed worldwide with over 20 peer reviewed articles [2].

The need for standardization was recognized early by the leaders in the field of TORS for OSA, and in 2014 a benchmark landmark publication was put forward

C. Vicini, M.D. • F. Montevecchi, M.D. (✉)
Head and Neck Department - ENT & Oral Surgery Unit - G.B. Morgagni - L. Pierantoni Hospital, Forlì – Infermi Hospital, Faenza - ASL of Romagna, Italy
e-mail: claudio@claudiovicini.com; filo651@hotmail.com; filippomontevecchi72@gmail.com

A. Campanini, M.D.
Head and Neck Department—ENT & Oral Surgery Unit,
G.B. Morgagni—L. Pierantoni Hospital, ASL of Romagna, Forlì, Italy

Infermi Hospital, ASL of Romagna, Faenza, Italy

I. Dallan, M.D.
First ENT Unit, Azienda Ospedaliero-Universitaria Pisana, Via Paradisa, 2, 56126 Pisa, Italy

Head and Neck Surgery & Forensic Dissection Research Center (HNS & FDRC), Department of Biotechnology and Life Sciences (DBSV), University of Insubria, Varese, Italy

P.T. Hoff, M.S., M.D. • M.E. Spector, M.D.
Department of Otolaryngology – Head and Neck Surgery,
University of Michigan Health System, Ann Arbor, MI 48109, USA

E.R. Thaler, M.D., F.A.C.S.
Division of General Otolaryngology, Head and Neck Surgery, Department of Otolaryngology-Head and Neck Surgery, University of Pennsylvania School of Medicine, Philadelphia, PA, USA

© Springer International Publishing Switzerland 2016

C. Vicini et al. (eds.), *TransOral Robotic Surgery for Obstructive Sleep Apnea*,
DOI 10.1007/978-3-319-34040-1_16

representing the results on seven centers examining the clinical outcomes of 243 patients undergoing TORS with or without multilevel surgery [2]. This publication represented an international experience with TORS for OSA, and allowed the examination of the clinical outcomes to be performed on a larger scale. These clinical outcomes are divided into two main areas for patients undergoing TORS for obstructive sleep apnea: safety of the procedure, which include the short-term and long-term complications, and efficacy of the procedure. This chapter will examine the expected outcomes for both the safety and efficacy of TORS in patients with obstructive sleep apnea.

16.2 Safety

Establishing the safety of a novel procedure is important to give both patients and surgeons the ability to provide proper counseling about the expected risk that each party is undertaking. The safety of trans-oral robotic surgery was first established by Weinstein and colleagues in cadaver and canine models [3, 4] and then further confirmed in multi-center clinical trials [5]. The approval for TORS was initially for oropharyngeal cancer, and it wasn't until 2009 the technology was approved for benign disease [6].

Transoral robotic surgery for obstructive sleep apnea has a unique set of risks, benefits, and complications compared to cancer patients. Patient goals in surgery for OSA are focused on quality of life rather than cancer cure, and the short- and long-term complications, although important in both benign and malignant disease, are the only primary outcome in patients with obstructive sleep apnea. Therefore the minimization of complications and long-term side effects are of the utmost importance.

J. Ahn, M.D.
Department of Otolaryngology – Head and Neck Surgery,
Columbia University Medical Center, New York, NY, USA
e-mail: jeffreyahn@gmail.com

P.M. Baptista, M.D., Ph.D.
Department of ORL, Clinica Universidad de Navarra,
Pamplona, Spain
e-mail: peterbaptista@gmail.com

M. Remacle, M.D., Ph.D. • G. Lawson, M.D.
Department of ORL-Head & Neck Surgery, Louvain University
Hospital of Mont Godinne, Therasse Avenue 1, 5530 Yvoir, Belgium
e-mail: remacle.marc@chl.lu; georges.lawson@uclouvain.be

M. Benazzo, M.D., Ph.D. • P. Canzi, M.D.
Department of Otolaryngology, IRCCS Policlinico San Matteo,
University of Pavia, 27100 Pavia, Italy
e-mail: m.benazzo@smatteo.pv.it; pcanzio@hotmail.com

Table 16.1 ASA Classification System: six-category physical status classification system defining an individual's overall functional status

Class	Definition
I	Healthy person
II	Mild systemic disease
III	Severe systemic disease
IV	Severe systemic disease that is a constant threat to life
V	A moribund person who is not expected to live without the operation
VI	A declared brain-dead person whose organs are being removed for donor purposes

ASA American Society of Anesthesiologists

Table 16.2 Complications of transoral robotic lingual tonsillectomy ± directed multilevel procedures

Complications	Vicini et al.	Glazer et al.	Hoff et al.
Bleeding	5.0 %	7.2 %	4.1 %
Dehydration/dysphagia	NR	9.6 %	9.9 %
Aspiration	NR	0.6 %	2.0 %
Readmission rate	NR	15 %	9.6 %
Total complications	21.5 %	24.7 %	20.1 %

NR not reported

Another complicating factor in treating patients with OSA with surgery is that obstructive sleep apnea patients typically have multiple other comorbidities, which can make surgical risks higher in these patients as well. Hoff and colleagues performed a multicenter review looking at the safety and feasibility of TORS in OSA in 285 patients, and noted that 22 % of patients had two or more comorbidities and 30 % of patients were American Society of Anesthesiology Classification 3 [7, 8] (Table 16.1). The use of a preoperative general medicine clinic may improve patient selection to decrease complication rates [9].

There have been three large reviews that have focused on complication rates in the immediate postoperative period [2, 7, 9]. Table 16.2 shows combined data from Vicini et al., Hoff et al., and Glazer et al. looking at complication rates in patients undergoing TORS for OSA. Glazer and colleagues divided the risk into major complications and minor complications, with major complications requiring a return trip to the operating room and minor complications typically self-limited [9]. The overall complication rate in these studies were 21.5 %, 24.7 % and 20.1 %.

These complication rates are similar to those reported in the literature, although there are no exact comparisons for TORS with multilevel surgery. Woodson and colleagues reported on a midline glossectomy technique, and the overall complication rate was 27 % [10]. Similarly, Hou et al. reported a complication rate of 24 % with midline glossectomy and uvulopalatopharyngoplasty [11]. Both of these studies included bleeding and dysphagia/odynophagia in their review. A large review of readmissions after tonsillectomy showed an emergency room readmission rate of

10.7 % and a hospital readmission rate of 1.8 %. Patients whose indication for surgery was sleep apnea and tonsillitis also had a 1.7 times increased risk of readmission in this study, consistent with the readmission rate in Glazer et al. and Hoff et al. [12].

While dysphagia and odynophagia are quite common after TORS for OSA, patients are allowed to have a normal diet quite quickly, and this is a self-limited problem. In the multicenter review by Vicini et al., a soft oral diet was tolerated by the majority of patients after 1 day, ranging from 1 to 4 days. The recovery of swallowing is supported by the lack of change in the 3 month BMI measurements performed in conjunction with the sleep study [2]. The mean preoperative and postoperative BMI for patients treated by Vicini and colleagues was 28.53 and 28.4, respectively.

Long-term changes of swallowing and taste disturbances are seldom reported. Vicini did report transient hypoguesia in 14 % of patients, with recovery of this in 8 months [2]. No patients underwent formal testing of taste measures. There was one patient who required a g-tube in the study by Glazer et al., which was removed later after speech and swallow therapy [9]. More research is needed into formal swallowing measurements to determine the long lasting effects on swallowing function.

Short- and long-term swallowing function has been analyzed by Eesa et al. [13]. In this study, 78 patients underwent TORS multilevel surgery including lingual tonsillectomy and supraglottoplasty. The MD Anderson Dysphagia Index (MDADI) was used to grade the degree of swallowing dysfunction. At short-term follow-up (1 week), 5 patients (6 %) demonstrated aspiration on gastrografin swallow, although none required gastric feeding tube. Long term (mean 20 ± 7 months) there were no patients with subjective complaints or requiring feeding tube.

Hoff et al. [7] completed a multicenter, retrospective cohort study in 2014 that demonstrated the safety of this procedure, which subsequently lead the FDA to grant approval for TORS benign base of tongue resection (BBOTR). This endorsement by the FDA did not include an approval for OSA; approval of TORS for moderate to severe OSA is pending further prospective data. Approval for TORS BBOTR in the USA has allowed surgeons to move forward; surgeons in other countries should be aware of their national regulatory environment.

16.3 Efficacy

The efficacy of transoral robotic surgery for obstructive sleep apnea has been defined in multiple ways. The objective measure of efficacy is most well-defined as the postoperative AHI obtained between 3 and 6 months after surgery. Compared to preoperative, almost all patients see reduction in their apnea hypopnea index (AHI), as seen in two large series of patients performed by Vicini et al. and Hoff et al. [2, 14]. The average reduction of the preoperative to postoperative AHI in these studies decreased by a rate of 48 % and 59 %, respectively. These improvements in AHI were seen in over 80 % of patients in both groups. Most patients, however, are not looking just to improve their AHI, rather they would like to come off CPAP altogether. Therefore, a close comparison to the literature looking at rates of success and cure from sleep

Table 16.3 Improvement, success, and cure rates in transoral robotic lingual tonsillectomy ± directed multilevel procedures

Rates	Vicini et al.	Hoff et al.	Thaler et al.
Improvement	NR	84 %	60%[a]
Success	67 %	51 %	45 %
Cure	23 %	14 %	NR

[a]Thaler et al. reports response rate instead of improvement, defined as >50 % reduction in preoperative AHI. Success in defined by >50 % reduction in AHI and AHI <20. Cure is defined as AHI <5. *NR* not reported

apnea altogether is necessary to make meaningful comparisons. The definition of success for obstructive sleep apnea has traditionally been defined as a decrease in the AHI by 50 % of baseline and AHI <20 and cure has been defined as AHI <5 [15, 16]. While we will first review the literature using these standards, there are probably other meaningful comparisons that need to be examined which we will discuss at the end of this section. TORS for OSA remains in its infancy therefore it is important to note that studies evaluating long-term efficacy have not been published.

The three largest retrospective reviews of outcomes looking at success and cure rates have been performed by Vicini et al., Hoff et al., and Thaler et al. [2, 14, 17]. The data on success and cure rates are shown in Table 16.3. These three articles all use transoral robotic surgery coupled with other multilevel surgery to treat obstructive sleep apnea. The overall success rates in these three studies were between 45–67 %. These results were stratified by preoperative risk factors, and prior surgery, as well as BMI greater than 30, and were found to be associated with worse outcomes [14, 17]. In fact, patients with BMI <25 seemed to be the best candidates for surgery, with a success rate of 78 %. Alternatively, patients who had prior surgery for their sleep apnea had a success rate of only in 30 % in the study by Thaler et al., making them a more cautious candidate for surgery.

While patients may not see a meaningful reduction in their AHI (not meeting criteria for success or cure), there are other metrics that require further research. There may be a change in the ratio of apneas to hypopneas within the AHI that could have clinical significance. In addition, the Epworth sleep scale, a validated questionnaire given to patients to determine their general level of daytime sleepiness, is typically given to these patients, but not used to determine levels of success or cure. For example, Thaler et al. reports an improvement of the ESS scores from 12.8 to 5.8 in 31 patients treated with TORS and multilevel surgery. This certainly means patients are feeling better regarding their daytime sleepiness, with a quantifiable result to consider the withdrawal of PAP therapy.

A final argument that can be made for considering the overall reduction in AHI and symptoms with achieving cure is that the majority of patients included in these studies have failed or noncompliant with PAP therapy. In this patient population, the reduction of AHI and improvement of subjective symptoms may mitigate the risks of the procedure as they have no other options for improvement. Maurer et al. showed that actual CPAP compliance can be as low as 60 % [18]. The adjusted AHI in patients using CPAP on an intermittent basis throughout the night is much worse than the reported sleep laboratory AHI; an adjusted AHI of 15 in patients using CPAP is similar to the results found in the large multicenter trial where 50 % of patients had and AHI <15 [2]. In highly selected patients we may be approaching equivalence with PAP for the primary treatment of OSA [19].

Other measures of success have been proposed including physiologic correction of systolic hypertension, improvement in mean O_2 saturation, oxygen desaturation index (ODI), and subjective quality of life measures including the Functional Outcome of Sleepiness Questionnaire (FOSQ) and Thornton snoring scale. There has also been a movement toward redefining success as an AHI of 15 rather than 20. Others question whether the weighting of apnea and hypopnea should be equivalent especially as we move toward home Type 2 and 3 sleep studies where accurate assessment of hypopnea is variable. Hobson showed that the success rate for OSA surgery can vary from 38.9 % to 91.7 % depending on the definition of apnea and hypopnea and the inclusion of reduction of AHI from preoperative values [20].

Ultimately the definition of success will have to be a combination of measures acceptable to both the sleep medicine community and the sleep surgery community. A unified definition of success will decrease conflicting statements that only serve to confused the ultimate consumer of this information—our patients.

References

1. Vicini C, Dallan I, Canzi P, Frassineti S, La Pietra MG, Montevecchi F. Transoral robotic tongue base resection in obstructive sleep apnoea-hypopnoea syndrome: a preliminary report. ORL J Otorhinolaryngol Relat Spec. 2010;72(1):22–7.
2. Vicini C, Montevecchi F, Campanini A, Dallan I, Hoff PT, Spector ME, Thaler E, Ahn J, Baptista P, Remacle M, Lawson G, Benazzo M, Canzi P. Clinical outcomes and complications associated with TORS for OSAHS: a benchmark for evaluating an emerging surgical technology in a targeted application for benign disease. ORL J Otorhinolaryngol Relat Spec. 2014;76(2):63–9. doi:10.1159/000360768. Epub 2014 Apr 23.
3. Hockstein NG, O'Malley Jr BW, Weinstein GS. Assessment of intraoperative safety in transoral robotic surgery. Laryngoscope. 2006 Feb;116(2):165–8.
4. Hockstein NG, Weinstein GS, O'malley Jr BW. Maintenance of hemostasis in transoral robotic surgery. ORL J Otorhinolaryngol Relat Spec. 2005;67(4):220–4. Epub 2005 Sept 5.
5. Weinstein GS, O'Malley Jr BW, Magnuson JS, Carroll WR, Olsen KD, Daio L, Moore EJ, Holsinger FC. Transoral robotic surgery: a multicenter study to assess feasibility, safety, and surgical margins. Laryngoscope. 2012 Aug;122(8):1701–7. doi:10.1002/lary.23294. Epub 2012 July 2.
6. Weinstein G, O'Malley Jr BW. FDA clears transoral robotic surgery—developed at Penn—for tumors of mouth, throat and voice box. 2009. http://www.uphs.upenn.edu/news/News_Releases/2009/12/rors-robotic head-neck-surgery/.
7. Hoff PT, D'Agostino MA, Thaler ER. Transoral robotic surgery in benign diseases including obstructive sleep apnea: safety and feasibility. Laryngoscope. 2015;125(5):1249–53. doi:10.1002/lary.25026. Epub 2014 Nov 12.
8. American Society of Anesthesiologists. ASA physical status classification system. Available at: http://www.asahq.org/Home/For-Members/Clinical-Information/ASA-Physical-Status-Classification-System. Accessed 22 Feb 2014.

9. Glazer TA, Hoff PT, Spector ME. Transoral robotic surgery for obstructive sleep apnea: perioperative management and postoperative complications. JAMA Otolaryngol Head Neck Surg. 2014;140(12):1207–12.
10. Woodson BT, Fujita S. Clinical experience with lingualplasty as part of the treatment of severe obstructive sleep apnea. Otolaryngol Head Neck Surg. 1992;107:40–8.
11. Hou J, Yan J, Wang B, et al. Treatment of obstructive sleep apneahypopnea syndrome with combined uvulopalatopharyngoplasty and midline glossectomy: outcomes from a 5-year study. Respir Care. 2012;57:2104–10.
12. Seshamani M, Vogtmann E, Gatwood J, et al. Prevalence of complications from adult tonsillectomy and impact on health care expenditures. Otolaryngol Head Neck Surg. 2014;150(4):574–81. doi:10.1177/0194599813519972.
13. Eesa M, Montevecchi F, Hendawy E, D'Agostino G, Meccariello G, Vicini C. Swallowing outcome after TORS for sleep apnea: short- and long-term evaluation. Eur Arch Otorhinolaryngol. 2015;272(6):1537–41. doi:10.1007/s00405-014-3480-x. Epub 2015 Jan 4.
14. Hoff PT, Glazer TA, Spector ME. Body mass index predicts success in patients undergoing transoral robotic surgery for obstructive sleep apnea. ORL J Otorhinolaryngol Relat Spec. 2014;76(5):266–72. doi:10.1159/000368415. Epub 2014 Nov 20.
15. Caples S, Rowley J, Prinsell J, et al. Surgical modifications of the upper airway for obstructive sleep apnea in adults: a systemic review and meta-analysis. Sleep. 2010;33:1396–407.
16. Elshaug AG, Moss JR, Southcott AM, Hiller JE. Redefining success in airway surgery for obstructive sleep apnea: a meta-analysis and synthesis of the evidence. Sleep. 2007;30:461–7.
17. Thaler ER, Rassekh CH, Lee JM, Weinstein GS, O'Malley Jr BW. Outcomes for multilevel surgery for sleep apnea: Obstructive sleep apnea, transoral robotic surgery, and uvulopalatopharyngoplasty. Laryngoscope. 2015;126:266. doi:10.1002/lary.25353 [Epub ahead of print].
18. Maurer JT, Verse T, Stuck BA, Hein G, Hörmann K. Surgery or nCPAP for OSA: response adjusted for compliance. Otolaryngol Head Neck Surg. 2002;127:66.
19. Rotenberg BW, Theriault J, Gottesman S. Redefining the timing of surgery for obstructive sleep apnea in anatomically favorable patients. Laryngoscope. 2014;124 Suppl 4:S1–9. doi:10.1002/lary.24720. Epub 2014 May 27.
20. Hobson JC, Robinson S, Antic NA, McEvoy RD, Windler S, Mackay S, Carney AS. What is "success" following surgery for obstructive sleep apnea? The effect of different polysomnographic scoring systems. Laryngoscope. 2012;122(8):1878–81. doi:10.1002/lary.23342. Epub 2012 May 7.

Chapter 17
Complication Management

Filippo Montevecchi, Saleh Ali AlGhamdi, and Chiara Bellini

17.1 Introduction

The first robotic OSAHS surgery was performed in 2008 and the first series outlining surgical affects was published in 2010 [1]. To date, an estimated 1200 trans-oral robotic surgery(s) (TORS) for OSAHS have been performed worldwide and a multicenter retrospective analysis of results and complications from seven academic centers has been published [2]. The purpose of this chapter is to analyze the possible complications that may occur during TORS for OSAHS.

17.2 Preoperative Assessment

Before undergoing any surgical treatment for OSAHS, patients should have a thorough anesthetic assessment to identify and manage those who are at high risk secondary to medical comorbidities. There is a long list of illnesses associated with OSAHS including treatment-resistant hypertension, dysrhythmias, pulmonary

F. Montevecchi, M.D. (✉)
Head and Neck Department - ENT & Oral Surgery Unit - G.B. Morgagni - L. Pierantoni Hospital, Forlì – Infermi Hospital, Faenza - ASL of Romagna, Italy
e-mail: filo651@hotmail.com; filippomontevecchi72@gmail.com

S.A. AlGhamdi, M.D.
ENT Department, King Fahd Armed Forces Hospital, Jeddah, Kingdom of Saudi Arabia
e-mail: alhajis7@yahoo.com

C. Bellini, M.D.
Head and Neck Department—ENT & Oral Surgery Unit, G.B. Morgagni—L. Pierantoni Hospital, ASL of Romagna, Forlì, Italy

Infermi Hospital, ASL of Romagna, Faenza, Italy
e-mail: chiarabe@inwind.it

© Springer International Publishing Switzerland 2016

C. Vicini et al. (eds.), *TransOral Robotic Surgery for Obstructive Sleep Apnea*,
DOI 10.1007/978-3-319-34040-1_17

hypertension, obesity, and metabolic syndrome [3, 4]. These conditions need to be optimized before surgical intervention. OSAHS, as a disorder in itself, is associated with an increased perioperative risk and postoperative surgical complications and this risk needs to also be considered prior to any intervention. Additionally, TORS for OSAHS is a BMI-sensitive procedure [5, 6]. In patients with BMI>30 the expected success rate decreases in accordance with an increasing BMI. Patient may benefit from a medically assisted weight loss program prior to any surgical intervention.

An important issue to consider in OSAHS surgery is the airway itself. In sleep apnea surgery, an already difficult airway can be further compromised by edema and bleeding. Difficult intubation facilities must be accessible and an endoscopic assisted intubation will often be necessary [7, 8]. Reintubation for postoperative edema or bleeding can be very difficult and the need for a tracheostomy should be considered whenever required. In our department (ENT Department, Morgagni-Pierantoni Hospital, Forlì, Italy), we recommend an elective tracheostomy for severe OSAHS cases especially if multi-level surgery is undertaken and the patient present difficult intubation [9, 10]. Mild to moderate OSAHS cases who are having limited surgery, have reasonably good airway anatomy, and have limited medical comorbidities do not need a routine tracheostomy. However, each patient is discussed on a case-by-case scenario with the surgical and anesthetic team before a final decision is reached. An additional and very important advantage in having a tracheostomy is that there is no tube obstructing the surgical view. This can be a significant advantage in a very narrow pharynx. Furthermore, with a tracheostomy in place it is possible to remove tongue base and epiglottis without any risk of compromising the upper airway due to edema and bleeding.

17.3 Intraoperative Complications

The knowledge of trans-oral anatomy is essential for avoiding intraoperative complications especially to the neurovascular bundle. During the TORS resection, magnification of up to 10× combined with a 3D image allows excellent visualization for identification of vessels and nerves. After the initial step of removal of the lingual tonsils from the base of tongue, additional muscle resection may be required to obtain an adequate anteroposterior sized airway and this should be done carefully under sufficiently high magnification. It is important to adjust the robotic scope appropriately, zooming in and out, to maintain this magnification. It is of paramount importance to maintain orientation using the tongue base midline as the point of reference to minimize risk to the hypoglossal nerve, lingual artery, and lingual neural branches. Due to the inherent anatomic variability of the tongue base and tissue distortion from tongue retraction and mouth gag placement, precise localization of these structures is not possible. Thus, an understanding of their anatomical course and landmarks is especially important.

17.3.1 *Anatomical Consideration*

The lingual artery arises from the external carotid artery at the level of the hyoid bone. It courses lateral to the middle constrictor muscle where it is crossed by the hypoglossal nerve, and then it passes deep to the hyoglossus muscle where it runs on the superior surface of the hyoid bone. It is in this location that it is vulnerable to injury during trans-oral base of tongue surgery. The lingual artery then gives off a suprahyoid branch, a dorsal lingual artery which passes to the dorsum of the tongue, the sublingual artery, and the arteria profunda linguae which passes between the genioglossus muscle and the inferior intrinsic tongue musculature. These arteries anastomose richly with their partners from the opposite side. The tongue is drained by lingual veins that pass to the internal jugular vein directly or via the facial and retromandibular veins.

The tongue receives motor supply from the hypoglossal nerve. The hypoglossal nerve emanates from the hypoglossal canal and descends behind the internal carotid artery and the glossopharyngeal nerve and vagus nerve. It then passes between the internal carotid artery and internal jugular vein, runs in front of the vagus nerve, and loops in front of the internal and external carotid artery and lingual artery. A small branch of the occipital artery feeding the sternocleidomastoid muscle crosses over the hypoglossal nerve just below the posterior belly of the digastric muscle. The nerve then passes over the hyoglossus muscle and runs along the superior border of the hyoid bone, deep to the digastric and mylohyoid muscles. It is here that the nerve is at most risk during trans-oral base of tongue surgery. The hypoglossal nerve divides into terminal branches that continue between the mylohyoid and genioglossus muscles. The posterior tongue receives predominant sensory innervation by the lingual branch of the glossopharyngeal nerve for both afferent sensation and taste [11–14].

17.3.2 *Bleeding/Hemostasis*

A vessel clip applier and an insulated bipolar forceps should be readily available throughout the surgery. The bipolar forceps needs to have an angled tip to achieve adequate access. This can allow the bedside assistant to manage intraoperative bleeding. As a 30° upward-facing scope is utilized during the procedure, all the non-robotic instruments should be angled, especially the suction devices that are used to suction smoke, blood, and provide counter-traction.

At the end of the procedure the wound is inspected carefully for hemostasis, and cautery or vessel clips are used as needed for persistent bleeding. A surface tissue hemostatic agent such as Tisseel® Fibrin Sealant® (Baxter, Deerfield, IL) can be applied in a thin layer, which some clinicians feel may also help with postoperative discomfort. The tongue and airway are inspected for edema at the end of the procedure to assess the possibility of an early tube removal or the necessity of a prolonged intubation or tracheostomy.

17.3.3 Intra-oral Trauma

An important intraoperative complication is dental or mouth trauma. To avoid damage to the teeth, the upper dental arch is protected with either a standard rubber tooth guard or a custom guard fabricated in the operating room from Aquaplast®. To avoid trauma to the oral cavity and oropharynx mucosa, the robotic instruments must be inserted under direct vision initially and then via the slave screen when it is no longer possible to visualize them trans-orally.

17.4 Immediate Postoperative Complications

The immediate postoperative period is crucial to avoid serious complications and the patient should be monitored carefully in a high-acuity nursing setting. Intravenous steroids are given to minimize lingual edema and nausea. Intravenous broad-spectrum antibiotics are infused pre- and postoperatively as per hospital protocol or surgeon preference to avoid possible infections.

If the patient did not undergo tracheostomy as the initial step in the operative procedure, the patient should have a prolonged postoperative intubation either in recovery or in an intensive care setting. This is done to avoid laryngospasm that may result from aspiration of saliva or blood. In an already difficult airway, reintubation is made even more difficult due to postoperative edema, bleeding, and modified anatomy. Prior to removal of the endotracheal tube, we check the airway with a flexible endoscope. This optimizes the timing of tube removal and is usually a few hours after the surgery. In the USA, patients are usually extubated in the operating room and observed overnight in the ICU or in a setting with cardiopulmonary monitoring and skilled nursing.

As detailed previously, in our institute, for patients with severe OSAHS, severe comorbid conditions, and a narrow mouth opening or other anatomical features suggesting a difficult intubation and reintubation a planned tracheostomy is recommended for post-op ventilation assistance, especially if multi-level surgery is scheduled. Among the above-quoted reasons for a preventive tracheostomy, the key one is the degree of difficulty for reintubation in case of postsurgical airway edema or postoperative bleeding.

During the first postoperative night, patients should be monitored in a high-acuity setting. In most institutions this would be in an intensive care or high dependency unit rather than the typical postoperative hospital ward. The patient should have continuous pulse oximetry and suction should be available at all times by the bedside and should be watched closely for bleeding and respiratory depression.

We find that many patients can swallow liquids comfortably without aspiration within a day of surgery, but this can vary considerably between patients. In our institution, we routinely do not insert a feeding tube and a liquid diet is started on postoperative day 1. We also continue oral steroids post-discharge on a tapering dose. Narcotics are used as needed, but this must be in the context of close observation of respiratory rate and level of consciousness, as recommended postoperatively for other OSAHS surgical procedures.

The length of stay can vary considerably depending upon a number of variables and surgeon comfort level. Tracheostomy by itself necessitates a multi-day hospital stay. Other determinants include the extent of surgery, comorbidities, pain control, and swallowing ability. In the USA, patient is discharged on the first postoperative day. However, in Europe, a longer hospitalization of 3–5 days is followed.

17.5 Delayed Postoperative Complications

Patients are followed closely after discharge. Diet is normalized as the healing progresses and formal therapist-directed swallowing therapy is rarely needed. Most patients will resume a normal diet within 1 month of surgery. Patients who have undergone multi-level surgery may need longer time than patients who have had only one site treated.

In case of delayed postoperative bleeding, if conservative measures fail, a suspension laryngoscope should be used to achieve an operative view of the base of tongue. It is unlikely that a view of the bleeding area will be achieved with a tonsil gag. Typically a suction-monopolar diathermy device is then used for hemostasis.

Another important and difficult-to-manage long-term complication is that of a synechia formation or stenosis of the oro-hypopharynx following TORS. If adequate exposure is not achieved at the time of TORS, and there is no sufficient space between tongue base epiglottis and the posterior pharyngeal wall, it is possible to injure the mucosa of the posterior and lateral oropharyngeal walls through the use of monopolar cautery. This circumferential damage could produce a concentric scar in the first months after surgery. This complication may necessitate long-term tracheostomy and gastrostomy tube. In order to avoid a concentric scar, especially in patients where a palate surgery is performed, a 1–2 cm strip of intact mucosa should be preserved between the palatine tonsil fossa and the tongue base. Pharyngeal stenosis is a devastating complication, so prevention is the best strategy.

17.6 Conclusion

The adverse events recorded as part of a multicentric study (seven centers among Europe and the USA) [2] are summarized. In 243 cases there was a 0.0 % mortality and a 20.5 % morbidity rate recorded, most of which are minor and of short term. The most common patient complaint was transient and mild hypogeusia (14.2 %), which recovered within 8 months in all the patients. Bleeding was the second most common complication (5 % of the procedures). In most of the cases (2.9 %) late postoperative bleeding was self-limited and did not require operative intervention. Only 1.7 % of the patients required an additional surgical procedure to control the bleeding. Finally, in 0.4 % of surgeries a significant intraoperative hemorrhage was reported. Pharyngeal scarring with minimal to mild stenosis was a late complication in 0.4 % of the procedures. Transient pharyngeal edema was observed in 0.4 % of patients.

In another study [15] the majority of patients experienced mild prolonged dysphagia and globus sensation. Their cohort experienced a 10 % revisit rate within the first 2 weeks after surgery. Readmission was primarily a result of uncontrolled pain and associated dehydration. In Europe patients are hospitalized for 3–5 days after surgery and dehydration is not an issue because the patients continue to receive intravenous crystalloid while hospitalized. In the USA patients were discharged on postoperative day 1, frequently without a feeding tube.

Overall, these series to date shows that there is a good side-effect profile for this procedure. It is generally well tolerated and complications are limited in number and severity. No deaths or definite severe impairment were registered. Complications are similar to those seen with other surgical treatments of OSA and minor complications such as globus sensation and dysgeusia improve within 6–8 months in most patients.

References

1. Vicini C, Dallan I, Canzi P, Frassineti S, La Pietra MG, Montevecchi F. Transoral robotic tongue base resection in obstructive sleep apnoea-hypopnoea syndrome: a preliminary report. ORL J Otorhinolaryngol Relat Spec. 2010;72(1):22–7.
2. Vicini C, Montevecchi F, Campanini A, et al. Clinical outcomes and complications associated with TORS for OSAHS in 243 patients. A benchmark for evaluating an emerging surgical technology in a targeted application for benign disease. ORL J Otorhinolaryngol Relat Spec. 2014;76(2):63–9 [Epub 2014 Apr 23].
3. Shahar E, Whitney CW, Redline S, et al. Sleep-disordered breathing and cardiovascular disease: cross-sectional results of the Sleep Heart Health Study. Am J Respir Crit Care Med. 2001;163(1):19–25.
4. Yaggi HK, Concato J, Kernan WN, Lichtman JH, Brass LM, Mohsenin V. Obstructive sleep apnea as a risk factor for stroke and death. N Engl J Med. 2005;353:2034–41.
5. Vicini C, Montevecchi F, Pang K, et al. Combined transoral robotic tongue base surgery and palate surgery in obstructive sleep apnea-hypopnea syndrome: Expansion sphincter pharyngoplasty versus uvulopalatopharyngoplasty. Head Neck. 2014;36:77–83.
6. Hoff PT, Glazer TA, Spector ME. Body mass index predicts success in patients undergoing transoral robotic surgery for obstructive sleep apnea. ORL J Otorhinolaryngol Relat Spec. 2014;76(5):266–72.
7. Kim JA, Lee JJ. Preoperative predictors of difficult intubation in patients with obstructive sleep apnea syndrome. Can J Anaesth. 2006;53(4):393–7.
8. Hillman DR, Loadsman JA, Platt PR, Eastwood PR. Obstructive sleep apnoea and anaesthesia. Sleep Med Rev. 2004;8(6):459–71.
9. Sun H, Lou W, Wang L, Wu Y. Clinical significance of preoperative tracheotomy in preventing perioperative OSAHS severe complications. Lin Chuang Er Bi Yan Hou Ke Za Zhi. 2005;19(9):394–5.

10. Campanini A, De Vito A, Frassineti S, Vicini C. Temporary tracheotomy in the surgical treatment of obstructive sleep apnea syndrome: personal experience. Acta Otorhinolaryngol Ital. 2003;23(6):474–8.
11. Moore EJ, Janus J, Kasperbauer J. Transoral robotic surgery of the oropharynx: clinical and anatomic considerations. Clin Anat. 2012;25(1):135–41. doi:10.1002/ca.22008. Review [Epub 2011 Nov 22].
12. Vicini C, Dallan I, Canzi P, et al. Transoral robotic surgery of the tongue base in obstructive sleep Apnea-Hypopnea syndrome: anatomic considerations and clinical experience. Head Neck. 2012;34(1):15–22.
13. Dallan I, Seccia V, Faggioni L, et al. Anatomical landmarks for transoral robotic tongue base surgery: comparison between endoscopic, external and radiological perspectives. Surg Radiol Anat. 2013;35(1):3–10. doi:10.1007/s00276-012-0983-2 [Epub 2012 May 29].
14. Lauretano AM, Li KK, Caradonna DS, Khosta RK, Fried MP. Anatomic location of the tongue base neurovascular bundle. Laryngoscope. 1997;107(8):1057–9.
15. Glazer TA, Hoff PT, Spector ME. Transoral robotic surgery for obstructive sleep apnea: perioperative management and postoperative complications. JAMA Otolaryngol Head Neck Surg. 2014;140(12):1207–12.

Chapter 18
Short- and Long-Term Dysphagia

Mohamed Eesa and Giuseppe Meccariello

18.1 Introduction

Deglutition is a complex event that is conventionally divided into an oral, pharyngeal, and esophageal phase. Normal deglutition requires fine neuromuscular coordination of the organs of the upper aerodigestive tracts. Particularly, the pharyngeal phase begins the involuntary part of the swallowing mechanism. The stimulus or stimuli that initiate the pharyngeal phase are not clearly defined, but appear to be derived from the end of the oral phase and are carried by the ninth and tenth cranial nerves to the swallowing center in the reticular substance of the upper medulla. The four key components of the pharyngeal phase are (1) closure of the nasopharynx to prevent nasal reflux by approximation of the soft palate to the posterior nasopharyngeal wall, (2) elevation and closure of the larynx, (3) contractions of the pharyngeal constrictors, and (4) opening of the cricopharyngeus muscle. As well known, surgical resection of head-neck cancer results in predictable pattern of dysphagia and aspiration [1, 2]. Nevertheless, swallowing capabilities are usually a questionable matter after performing transoral robotic surgery (TORS) either for malignancy or obstructive sleep apnea (OSA) [3–16].

M. Eesa, M.B., B.Ch.
Department of Otolaryngology and Head – Neck Surgery, University of Zagazig, Zagazig 44519, Sharkia, Egypt
e-mail: dr.eesaorl@gmail.com

G. Meccariello, M.D. (✉)
Head and Neck Department—ENT & Oral Surgery Unit, G.B. Morgagni—L. Pierantoni Hospital, ASL of Romagna, Forlì, Italy

Infermi Hospital, ASL of Romagna, Faenza, Italy
e-mail: drmeccariello@gmail.com

© Springer International Publishing Switzerland 2016

C. Vicini et al. (eds.), *TransOral Robotic Surgery for Obstructive Sleep Apnea*, DOI 10.1007/978-3-319-34040-1_18

18.2 Our Experience

The first robotic procedure for the treatment of sleep apnea was done in May 2008 at G.B. Morgagni- L. Pierantoni Hospital in Forlì. Since then, TORS is representing an important cornerstone for the surgical treatment of sleep apnea, especially in patients with the principal site of collapse in tongue base and epiglottis. In our clinical practice before TORS, we recommend to perform a drug-induced sedation endoscopy (DISE) in all patients with suspicious tongue base collapse in order to confirm the collapsible sites evaluated during an in-office endoscopy and to plan a multilevel surgery as described in Chap. 18. Unfortunately, besides the well-known postoperative dysphagia in oropharyngeal/laryngeal cancer patients, little is known about the possible implication on swallowing after sleep surgery. To better understand this important issue, we carried out a study [17] on 78 patients (57 males and 21 females) with mean 48 years/old (range 12–72 years/old) who underwent TORS for sleep apnea. The operative technique is already described in Chap. 25. The minimal sufficient tongue base tissue volume of 7 cm^3 is recommended for alleviating obstruction. In our study, larger number of patients underwent TORS for sleep apnea during the same period but we included only patients with available follow-up data. All patients were routinely evaluated on the swallowing functions with video fluoroscopic swallow study, and chest X-ray during the first postoperative week. Additional methods were applied for evaluating the swallowing function postoperatively including MD Anderson Dysphagia Inventory (MDADI) questionnaire [18] which the patient had to fill in a preoperative visit, during first week postoperatively and after 1 month post-surgery. Additional data about start of oral feeding (days), nasogastric feeding (days), and tracheal tube (days) were collected. Subjective complaints by the patients themselves were collected for the long-term evaluation. The patients were followed up for average period of 20 ± 7.12 months (range 7–32 months). Demographic and clinical data were recorded including patient age, sex, type of surgical procedures performed, TORS operative time, and volume of tissue removed.

Only 23 out of 78 underwent tongue base reduction alone, while the remaining 55 underwent TORS in combination with other procedures as a part of multilevel surgery. Epiglottoplasty was done in all cases (100 %). Tracheostomy was done in 64 (82 %) patients, while 13 (18 %) procedures were done without tracheostomy. Associated surgical procedures (nasal and/or palatal) were done in 70 % (55 of 78). Median anterior glossectomy was added in 19 % (15 of 78) patients to further reduce oral tongue (Table 18.1). The operative time calculated for TORS procedure alone ranged from 15 to 90 min with the mean of 39 ± 11 min. Calculation of the excised volume of tongue base and epiglottic tissue was routinely done and it ranged from 3 to 40 cm^3 with the mean of 12.35 ± 5.77 cm^3. The mean time of hospital stay was 8.5 ± 2.63 days (range 5–19 days). The mean time for tracheal tube removal was 3.5 days (range 3–4 days). The mean postoperative follow-up time was 20 ± 7.12 months (range 7–32 months). On short-term basis; various parameters

Table 18.1 Patient and treatment characteristics

Characteristics	No. (%)
Sex	
Male	57 (73)
Female	21 (17)
Associated procedures	
Tracheostomy	64 (82)
Nose and/or palate	55 (70)
Median anterior glossectomy	15 (19)
Epiglottoplasty	78 (100)

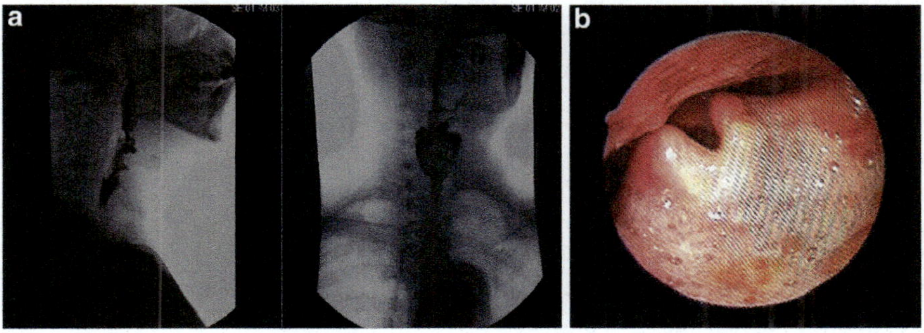

Fig. 18.1 (**a**) Video fluoroscopic swallow study after first postoperative week showing normal swallowing; (**b**) fiber-optic nasoendoscopy after 2 weeks of the same patient showing good healing with complete coverage of the removed part by mucosa

were used to evaluate swallowing outcomes in our patients, first using MDADI questionnaire which the patient had to fill in a preoperative visit, after first week postoperatively and after 1 month post-surgery. By comparing the preoperative score with the average of the two scores obtained postoperatively, there was minimal insignificant short-term impact on the swallowing function (4.58 ± 7.03 preoperative versus 5.18 ± 8.32 postoperative scores, $p=0.56$).

Considering the result of video fluoroscopic swallow study performed to the patients in the first postoperative week after removal of tracheal tube, we noticed 59 (76 %) patients with normal swallowing (Fig. 18.1), while 14 (18 %) patients showed minimal aspiration, but only 5 (6 %) patients experienced significant aspiration. Correlating the total volume of tissue removed from both tongue base and epiglottis to the results of video fluoroscopic swallow study regarding aspiration, no statistically significant relationship was observed ($p=0.72$) (Fig. 18.2). Furthermore, any significant correlations between results of video fluoroscopic swallow study regarding aspiration and the different procedures added to TORS, such as midline anterior glossectomy or palatal surgeries, were not found ($p=0.51$, $p=0.09$, respectively). Additional parameters used are:

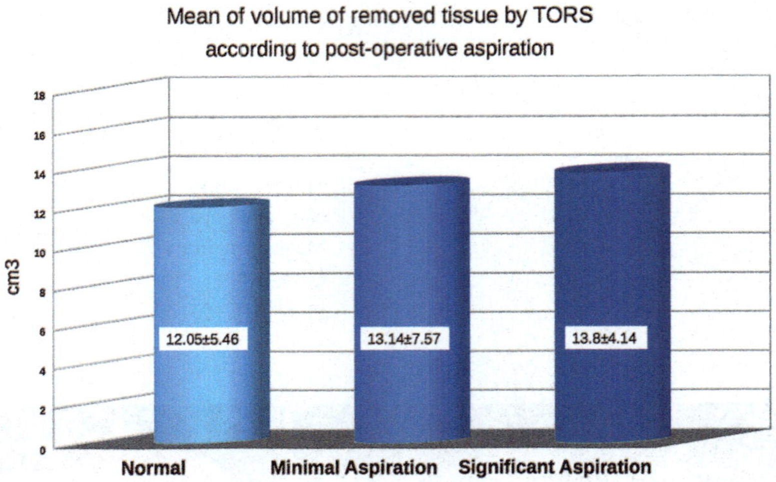

Fig. 18.2 Correlation among volumes of removed tissue from tongue base and epiglottis with grade of aspiration

- The timing for start of oral feeding: mean time 1.05 ± 0.25 days, range 1–3.
- Needing for nasogastric tube feeding: none of our patients needed nasogastric tube feeding.
- Finally, by evaluating chest X-ray findings as an indicator for chest problems related to aspiration: 72 (92 %) patients showed no lung infection or aspiration signs; 1 (1.2 %) patient showed irritation bronchitis and 1 (1.2 %) patient showed lung parenchymal density, possibly related to aspiration.

On long-term basis, none of all patients complained impairment of swallowing as assessed by the long-term consultations scheduled in the postoperative follow-up.

Moreover, by strictly following the 19 patients with initial abnormal findings on video fluoroscopic swallow study, we could demonstrate that their swallowing complaints disappeared completely within 3 months postoperatively and they also showed no remarkable weight loss related to their swallowing problems.

18.3 Discussion

One aim of this chapter is to describe the common problems related to swallowing that we usually encounter during our practice and to explain the evolution of these problems on long-term follow-up together with its impact on the patient quality of life. The results of our experience demonstrate no significant short-term impacts on swallowing in patients who underwent TORS for sleep apnea proved by nonsignificant increase in MDADI score after surgery. Also, by evaluating the results of video fluoroscopic swallow study that is usually performed in the first postoperative week, the percentage of significant aspiration was very low (6 %). Chest problems detected on chest X-ray and related to aspiration [irritation bronchitis (1.2 %) and lung parenchymal density (1.2 %)] are very low compared to the overall patient number. There was also rapid start of oral feeding within an average of 1–3 days with out needing of nasogastric feeding tube placement, but with a clear impact on shortening the hospital stay.

These results are not consistent with Richmon et al. [16] who stated that patients undergoing TORS for OSA are at greater risk of delay in initiation of oral diet and increased postoperative length of stay.

Also, they are better when compared to Chabolle's open tongue base reduction and hyoid epiglottopexy in which the start of oral feeding ranged from 9 to 21 days with mean of 15 days with decannulation range of 4–14 days and mean of 7 days [19].

Fujita et al. [20] reported on case of prolonged odynophagia after laser midline glossectomy and one case of minor change in taste, otherwise no persistent difficulties in swallowing. Mickelson et al. [21] reported no patients with prolonged or persistent dysphagia, odynophagia, loss of taste sensation, or aspiration after laser midline glossectomy. Powell et al. [22] stated that swallowing evaluations were unchanged from pretreatment and remained normal after radiofrequency tongue base reduction. De Vito et al. [23] did not report any significant complications with multilevel radiofrequency ablation including tongue base. Unfortunately, most of these studies did not provide real objective figures about swallowing problems after tongue base management.

We noticed that most of our patients experienced transient postoperative tongue numbness, and dysgeusia that is often described by the patients as altered sense of taste or a bitter/metallic taste. Fortunately, this complaint disappeared within 6 months in most of our patients (99 %) with only one patient (1 %) having persistent dysgeusia. We could notice also that irrespective of other associated procedures on the palate and even with performing tracheostomy, the final outcome is reasonable and the incidence of real and persistent dysphagia is very low, as we did not observe any significant and objective dysphagia after 6 months postoperatively especially by strictly following up the 19 patients with initial abnormal findings on video fluoroscopic swallow study. In five patients, where a subjective paresthesia in the pharyngeal area and in tongue base was registered, a completely normal physical examination, negative endoscopy, and a totally normal functional profile at swallowing protocol in our institution (fluoroscopy, functional endoscopic evaluation of swallowing) were evident. It means that a subjective subtle complaint must be put into account without any need of special therapy. One more additional observation in the analysis of our experience was the absence of any significant correlation between the incidence of aspiration problems as shown on video fluoroscopic swallow study and the volume of tissue removed from both tongue base and epiglottis. In our opinion, this will give more confidence during resection of tongue base but certainly with respect to the neural and vascular anatomy of that region.

In a previous unpublished data, we noticed that success is volume sensitive, and that was evident when we divided our patients into three groups (Fig. 18.3) according to the volume of tissue removed from both tongue base and epiglottis and calculated the percentage of successful and failed cases in each group, the group where between 10 and

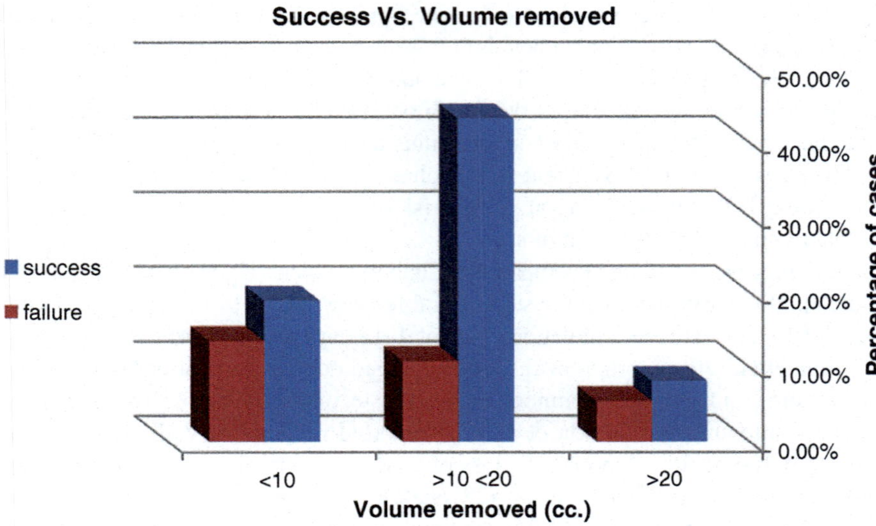

Fig. 18.3 Success versus volumes of removed tissue from tongue base and epiglottis

20 cm^3 of tissues were removed showed greater success-to-failure ratio, and accordingly we considered removal of 10–20 cm^3 as ideal for our resection in order to get better outcome after surgery.

18.4 Conclusion

- Transoral robotic surgery can be safely performed in OSA-suffering patients with an acceptable outcome.
- The return to normal oral feeding is rapid and complete with no negative impacts on quality of life.
- The postoperative swallowing assessment is highly recommended in order to identify the signs of aspiration.
- An early identification of swallowing impairment allows a quick and adequate restoring.

References

1. Walther EK. Dysphagia after pharyngolaryngeal cancer surgery: Part I. Pathophysiology of postsurgical deglutition. Dysphagia. 1995;10:275–8.
2. Kronenberger MB, Meyers AD. Dysphagia following head and neck cancer surgery. Dysphagia. 1994;9:236–44.

3. Sinclair CF, McColloch NL, Carroll WR, Rosenthal EL, Desmond RA, Magnuson JS. Patient-perceived and objective functional outcomes following transoral robotic surgery for early oropharyngeal carcinoma. Arch Otolaryngol Head Neck Surg. 2011;137:1112–6.
4. Moore EJ, Olsen KD, Kasperbauer JL. Transoral robotic surgery for oropharyngeal squamous cell carcinoma: a prospective study of feasibility and functional outcomes. Laryngoscope. 2009;119:2156–64.
5. Hurtuk A, Agrawal A, Old M, Teknos TN, Ozer E. Outcomes of transoral robotic surgery: a preliminary clinical experience. Otolaryngol Head Neck Surg. 2011;145:248–53.
6. Moore EJ, Olsen SM, Laborde RR, García JJ, Walsh FJ, Price DL, Janus JR, Kasperbauer JL, Olsen KD. Long-term functional and oncologic results of transoral robotic surgery for oropharyngeal squamous cell carcinoma. Mayo Clin Proc. 2012;87:219–25.
7. Kelly K, Johnson-Obaseki S, Lumingu J, Corsten M. Oncologic, functional and surgical outcomes of primary Transoral Robotic Surgery for early squamous cell cancer of the oropharynx: a systematic review. Oral Oncol. 2014;50:696–703.
8. Hutcheson KA, Holsinger FC, Kupferman ME, Lewin JS. Functional outcomes after TORS for oropharyngeal cancer: a systematic review. Eur Arch Otorhinolaryngol. 2015;272:463–71.
9. More YI, Tsue TT, Girod DA, Harbison J, Sykes KJ, Williams C, Shnayder Y. Functional outcomes following transoral robotic surgery vs primary chemoradiotherapy in patients with advanced-stage oropharynx and supraglottis cancers. JAMA Otolaryngol Head Neck Surg. 2013;139:43–8.
10. Van Abel KM, Moore EJ, Carlson ML, Davidson JA, Garcia JJ, Olsen SM, Olsen KD. Transoral robotic surgery using the thulium:YAG laser: a prospective study. Arch Otolaryngol Head Neck Surg. 2012;138:158–66.
11. Leonhardt FD, Quon H, Abrahao M, O'Malley Jr BW, Weinstein GS. Transoral robotic surgery for oropharyngeal carcinoma and its impact on patient-reported quality of life and function. Head Neck. 2012;34:146–54.
12. Iseli TA, Kulbersh BD, Iseli CE, Carroll WR, Rosenthal EL, Magnuson JS. Functional outcomes after transoral robotic surgery for head and neck cancer. Otolaryngol Head Neck Surg. 2009;141:166–71.
13. Weinstein GS, Quon H, Newman HJ, et al. Transoral robotic surgery alone for oropharynx cancer. Arch Otolaryngol Head Neck Surg. 2012;138:628–34.
14. Glazer TA, Hoff PT, Spector ME. Transoral robotic surgery for obstructive sleep apnea: perioperative management and postoperative complications. JAMA Otolaryngol Head Neck Surg. 2014;140:1207–12.
15. Vicini C, Montevechi F, Magnuson JS. Robotic surgery for obstructive sleep apnea. Curr Otorhinolaryngol Rep. 2013;1:130–6.
16. Richmon JD, Feng AL, Yang W, Starmer H, Quon H, Gourin CG. Feasibility of rapid discharge after transoral robotic surgery of the oropharynx. Laryngoscope. 2014;24:2518–25.
17. Eesa M, Montevecchi F, Hendawy E, D'Agostino G, Meccariello G, Vicini C. Swallowing outcome after TORS for sleep apnea: short- and long-term evaluation. Eur Arch Otorhinolaryngol. 2015;272:1537–41.
18. Chen AY, Frankowski R, Bishop-Leone J, Hebert T, Leyk S, Lewin J, Goepfert H. The development and validation of a dysphagia-specific quality-of-life questionnaire for patients with head and neck cancer: the M. D. Anderson dysphagia inventory. Arch Otolaryngol Head Neck Surg. 2001;127(7):870–6.
19. Chabolle F, Wagner I, Séquert C, Lachiver X, Coquille F, Fleury B, Blumen M. Tongue base reduction with hyoid epiglottoplasty. A surgical alternative in severe sleep apnea syndromes (in French). Ann Otolaryngol Chir Cervicofac. 1998;115:322–31.
20. Fujita S, Woodson BT, Clark JL, Wittig R. Laser midline glossectomy as a treatment for obstructive sleep apnea. Laryngoscope. 1991;101:805–9.
21. Mickelson SA, Rosenthal L. Midline glossectomy and epiglottidectomy for obstructive sleep apnea syndrome. Laryngoscope. 1997;107:614–9.

22. Powell NB, Riley RW, Guilleminault C. Radiofrequency tongue base reduction in sleep-disordered breathing: a pilot study. Otolaryngol Head Neck Surg. 1999;120:656–64.
23. De Vito A, Frassineti S, Panatta ML, Montevecchi F, Canzi P, Vicini C. Multilevel radiofrequency ablation for snoring and OSAHS patients therapy: long-term outcomes. Eur Arch Otorhinolaryngol. 2012;269:321–30.

Chapter 19
Failures Management

Claudio Vicini, Claudia Zanotti, L.B.L. Benoist, Gianluca Giorgio Marrano, and Nico de Vries

19.1 Introduction

Patients who undergo TORS for OSA are routinely scheduled for a control postoperative sleep study 6–9 months after the procedure as well as complete head and neck clinical evaluation, including awake fiberoptic examination of the upper airway. If the patient's data still meets the International Classification Systems of Disorders version 3 (ICSD-3) criteria for the diagnosis of OSA, and the patient is still eligible for CPAP according to Associazione Italiana di Pneumologia Ospedaliera (AIPO) Guidelines [1] the surgery outcome is considered as "failure", and a new complete work up is offered in order to understand why TORS failed and what other options are available.

C. Vicini, M.D. (✉)
Head and Neck Department - ENT & Oral Surgery Unit - G.B. Morgagni - L. Pierantoni Hospital, Forlì – Infermi Hospital, Faenza - ASL of Romagna, Italy
e-mail: claudio@claudiovicini.com

C. Zanotti, M.D. • G.G. Marrano, M.D.
Head and Neck Department—ENT & Oral Surgery Unit, G.B. Morgagni—L. Pierantoni Hospital, ASL of Romagna, Forlì, Italy

Infermi Hospital, ASL of Romagna, Faenza, Italy
e-mail: zanotti.claudia89@gmail.com; gianluca.giorgiomarrano@inwind.it

L.B.L. Benoist, M.D.
Department of Otolaryngology, OLVG Location West, Amsterdam, The Netherlands
e-mail: l.benoist@erasmusmc.nl

N. de Vries, M.D., Ph.D.
Department of Otolaryngology, OLVG Location West, Amsterdam, The Netherlands

Department of Otolaryngology, University of Antwerp, Antwerp, Belgium

© Springer International Publishing Switzerland 2016

C. Vicini et al. (eds.), *TransOral Robotic Surgery for Obstructive Sleep Apnea*,
DOI 10.1007/978-3-319-34040-1_19

19.2 Clinical Evaluation

In the typical history of most failures the patient and the bed partner describe an initial complete symptoms free interval of 2–4 months and after which there is a gradual and progressive recurrence of snoring, witnessed apneas, daytime sleepiness, nonrestorative sleep and fatigue. Despite worsening of symptoms following an initial improvement most patients do not have recurrence of choking and gasping episodes. In many cases patients also complain of mild persistent local side effects including: pharyngeal paresthesias, pharyngeal dryness, and subjective dysphagia.

Physical examination aims to provide a thorough assessment of the operated sites, which in most cases includes the nose, palate, tongue base, and supraglottis (multilevel surgery). This detailed examination includes the preoperative clinical findings, polysomnography, imaging data, as well as a description of the intraoperative findings, which includes recorded video imaging. Common reported clinical findings after surgical failure include:

1. Narrowing of the oropharyngeal inlet due to circular scar (this was only seen in LAUP or UPPP cases);
2. Very "high" tongue base (long distance between circumvallate papilla and epiglottis);
3. Insufficient tissue removal in the superior aspect of the tongue base, close to the circumvallate papilla.

19.3 Sleep Study

A careful analysis of the sleep study data is one more essential step in analysis of failures.

Surgical success was defined as a reduction of the AHI of greater than 50 % and an AHI below 15. Response—or partial effect—was defined as a reduction of the AHI greater than 50 % and below 20 [2]. In the great majority of the cases we noticed some typical profiles:

1. In the group of responders (AHI reduction greater than 50 % and less than 20), the overall number of events is reduced, but the sleep parameters including apnea hypopnea index (AHI) and oxygen desaturation index (ODI) do not fulfill the criteria for cure. Fortunately, we did not encounter cases of deterioration of sleep parameters (no case of postoperative AHI greater than preoperative AHI).
2. In the great majority of failures the ratio between apneas and hypopneas/RERAs was significantly reduced (more hypopneas/and RERAs, but less apneas).
3. If patients did not suffer from Positional OSA (POSA) before surgery, they very often became positional after TORS. In cases in which POSA was registered before surgery, it usually remained unchanged after surgery, albeit at a lower level of RDI. In (Fig. 19.1) a typical example is shown. Before surgery patient was affected by no positional OSA (AHI 70). After TORS, the AHI improved to 22.7, with a supine AHI of 48.2 (supine sleeping time = 44.3 % of total sleeping time, TST) and a non-supine AHI of 2.4 (not-supine sleeping time = 55.7 % of TST).

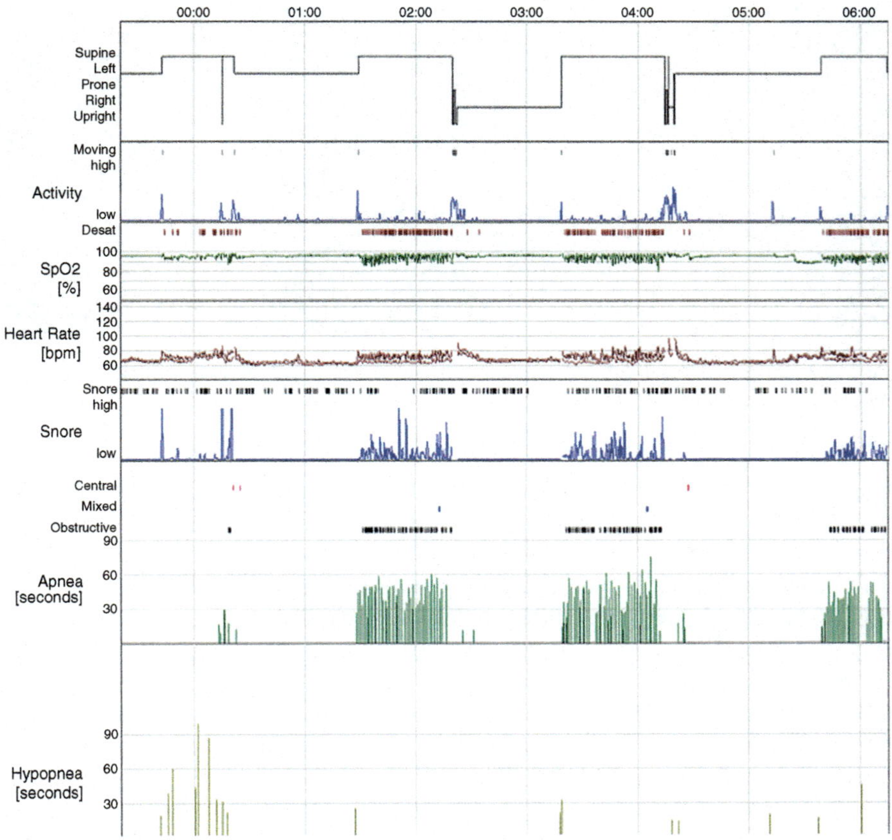

Fig. 19.1 Patient affected by POSA after TORS. Before surgery patient had no POSA. The sleep study after TORS shows clusters of apnea in supine position and absence of apnea in lateral position

19.4 Sleep Endoscopy

All surgical failures are scheduled for DISE. Imaging of the upper airway—CT scan or MRI—is included in the postoperative work-up. DISE is carried out according to the published protocol adopted at our Institutions, and in accordance to the DISE European Position Paper [3]. The DISE findings are scored according to the NOHL or VOTE classification system. In Fig. 19.2, preoperative and postoperative AHI was plotted against cumulative NOHL score in 27 failed cases. The steep course of the preoperative curve is due to the multisite obstructions in this group of patients, all of whom received a multilevel procedure (nose, palate, tongue base, supraglottis). The more horizontal line of postoperative data indicates that only one obstructing site remains and is likely responsible for the residual OSA. As shown, persistent obstruction at the palatal level is more common than residual obstruction at the

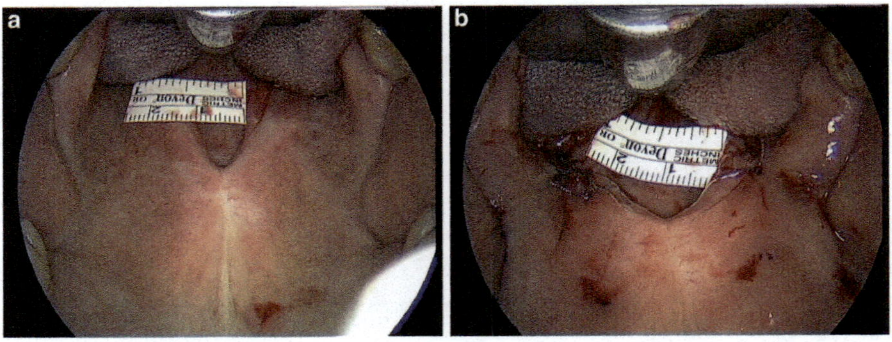

Fig. 19.2 (**a**) A LAUP carried out at another institution. (**b**) LAUP revised in BRP as part of a multilevel surgery for OSA including TORS

retro-lingual level (2:1 ratio). Residual obstruction occurred more often when UPPP was the palate procedure, as was performed in our first group of cases. The introduction of ESP and BRP [4, 5], not only proved to be more effective in reducing AHI, it furthermore reduced the percentage of failures related to residual palatal obstruction (unpublished data). In addition, failure was registered more commonly when surgery was performed by an inexperienced surgeon ($p<0.05$, unpublished data).

In residual collapse of the tongue base, DISE allows for recognition of different obstruction patterns. The most commonly observed obstruction pattern is a superior tongue base or oral tongue collapse in which the tongue strikes the soft palate causing secondary retro-palatal obstruction.

Less frequently, lateral tongue base instability is observed causing a concentric collapse of the tongue base resulting in an "in rolling" of the lateral parts of the tongue toward the midline.

19.5 Rescue Options

If the patient refuses a surgical revision, a conservative option can be offered and include:

Weight loss. Weight reduction is strongly recommended when the postoperative BMI exceeds the preoperative BMI. Typically TORS for OSA patients undergo a transitory weight loss following surgery, however most patients have returned to their preoperative level within 3 months. For those patients that exceed their preoperative weight nutrition counselling is recommended.

CPAP. Ventilation therapy is rarely accepted in this patient population. However, patients are counselled that after surgery the airway pressure may be reduced and their potential for CPAP compliance increased.

Oral Appliance therapy. Mandibular Advancement Devices (MAD) have proved to be of significant practical utility and the compliance is higher than CPAP. Patients with temporal-mandibular joint dysfunction or poor dentition may be not candidate for this type of therapy.

Positional therapy. In the last couple of years electronically assisted positional training with a new-generation smart positional therapy was introduced and applied in cases of residual POSA [6–8]. It has become apparent that while most patients with mild OSA are positional (their AHI is at least twice as high in supine position than in the other sleep positions), most cases with severe OSA are nonpositional. Since untreated OSA is a gradually progressive disease, mild OSA can deteriorate into moderate to severe or even extreme OSA. The phenomenon is reversible; a recent finding shows that after incomplete success by any methods, severe OSA can revert to moderate, or even mild POSA. In such cases the reduction of the AHI is more apparent in lateral position than in supine position. This trend has been observed after MAD therapy [9], weight loss by bariatric surgery [10], maxillo-mandibular advancement [11], and after UPPP [12]. A recent study in 33 cases of partially effective OSA surgery will be published shortly elsewhere (Benoist and De Vries, yet unpublished data). Adjunctive positional therapy as salvage after TORS/multilevel surgery can be of great value as well. In our Institutions we offered rescue Positional Therapy as an alternative to MAD. It was accepted by 50 % of the patients, with an efficacy rate of 80 %.

Revision surgery was offered as a first line of treatment and carried out in many cases of failure, mostly in the palatal area. Typically, UPPP failures demonstrated insufficient expansion of the retropalatal airway and medialization of the posterior pillars causing palatal stenosis. In most of these cases failed UPPP was salvaged using the technique of ESP or BRP.

In some cases of failed ESP, salvage could be obtained using BRP. To date we have had no failures following BRP. In Fig. 19.2a and b a LAUP carried out at another institution was subsequently revised as part of a multilevel surgery for OSA including TORS. A BRP was successfully performed. Revision surgery of the tongue base (additional TORS resection) has also been performed with less predictable results. If the area anterior to the circumvallate papilla (oral tongue) was the cause of failure, TORS anterior midline glossectomy was performed. Finally, hypoglossal nerve stimulators may offer one more tool for addressing residual tongue base collapse [13].

References

1. Italian AIPO guidelines.
2. Richard W, Kox D, den Herder C, van Tinteren H, de Vries N. One stage multilevel surgery (uvulopalatopharyngoplasty, hyoid suspension, radiofrequent ablation of the tongue base with/without genioglossus advancement), in obstructive sleep apnea syndrome. Eur Arch Otorhinolaryngol. 2006 Oct 25 [Epub ahead of print].
3. De Vito A, Carrasco Llatas M, Vanni A, Bosi M, Braghiroli A, Campanini A, de Vries N, Hamans E, Hohenhorst W, Kotecha BT, Maurer J, Montevecchi F, Piccin O, Sorrenti G, Vanderveken OM, Vicini C. European position paper on drug-induced sedation endoscopy (DISE). Sleep Breath. 2014;18(3):453–65. doi:10.1007/s11325-014-0989-6 [Epub 2014 May 26].

4. Vicini C, Montevecchi F, Pang K, Bahgat A, Dallan I, Frassineti S, et al. Combined transoral robotic tongue base surgery and palate surgery in obstructive sleep apnea-hypopnea syndrome: expansion sphincter pharyngoplasty versus uvulopalatopharyngoplasty. Head Neck. 2014;36(1):77–83.
5. Vicini C, Hendawy E, Campanini A, Eesa M, Bahgat A, AlGhamdi S, Montevecchi F, et al. Barbed reposition pharyngoplasty (BRP) for OSAHS: a feasibility, safety, efficacy and teachability pilot study. "We are on the giant's shoulders". Eur Arch Otorhinolaryngol. 2015;272(10):3065–70.
6. Ravesloot MJL, van Maanen JP, Dun L, de Vries N. The undervalued potential of positional therapy in position dependent snoring and obstructive sleep apnea—a review of the literature. Sleep Breath. 2013;17(1):39–49.
7. Van Maanen JP, Meester KAW, Dun LN, Koutsourelakis I, Witte BI, Laman DM, Hilgevoord AAJ, de Vries N. The Sleep Position trainer: a new treatment for positional obstructive sleep apnoea. Sleep Breath. 2013;17(2):771–9.
8. van Maanen JP, de Vries N. Long-term effectiveness and compliance of positional therapy with the sleep position trainer in the treatment of positional obstructive sleep apnea syndrome. Sleep. 2014;37(7):1209–15. doi:10.5665/sleep.3840.
9. Dieltjens M, Vroegop AV, Verbruggen AE, Wouters K, Willemen M, De Backer WA, Verbraecken JA, Van de Heyning PH, Braem MJ, de Vries N, Vanderveken OM. A promising concept of combination therapy for positional obstructive sleep apnea. Sleep Breath. 2014 Oct 22 [Epub ahead of print].
10. Morong S, Benoist LB, Ravesloot MJ, Laman DM, de Vries N. The effect of weight loss on OSA severity and position dependence in the bariatric population. Sleep Breath. 2014;18(4):851–6. doi:10.1007/s11325-014-0955-3 [Epub 2014 Mar 1].
11. Benoist LBL, de Ruiter MHT, de Lange J, de Vries N. Residual POSA after maxillomandibular advancement in patients with severe OSA. In: De Vries N, Ravesloot MJL, van Maanen JP, editors. Positional therapy in obstructive sleep apnea. New York: Springer; 2015. p. 312–30.
12. van Maanen JP, Witte BI, de Vries N. Theoretical approach towards increasing effectiveness of palatal surgery in obstructive sleep apnea: role for concomitant positional therapy? Sleep Breath. 2014;18(2):341–9. doi:10.1007/s11325-013-0891-7 [Epub 2013 Sep 7].
13. Strollo Jr PJ, Soose RJ, Maurer JT, de Vries N, Cornelius J, Froymovich O, Hanson RD, Padhya TA, Steward DL, Gillespie MB, Woodson BT, Van de Heyning PH, Goetting MG, Vanderveken OM, Feldman N, Knaack L, Strohl KP. STAR Trial Group. Upper-airway stimulation for obstructive sleep apnea. N Engl J Med. 2014;370(2):139–49.

Part IV
TORS for OSAS in Geographic Perspective: How to Run a Program in Different Countries

Chapter 20
The North American Experience

Paul T. Hoff, Robson Capasso, and Umamaheswar Duvvuri

20.1 Introduction

The birthplace of TORS for OSA resides in Forli, Italy. Many of the early adapters of this technique travelled to Italy and were mentored by Dr. Vicini and Montevecchi. The Forli approach to patients with OSA incorporates careful office assessment and also incorporated drug-induced sedated endoscopy (DISE) early in their experience. For the many who have adopted TORS as part of their armamentarium for the treatment of OSA, the environment in North America (USA) has allowed many centers to flourish, each with its own unique experiences. In general the early programs have either centered in large academic institutions or in a handful of private practice community hospitals eager to apply this new technology.

Surgeons interested in TORS in 2015 are at a distinct advantage compared to the early adapters, as much of the groundwork has been completed. The work by Vicini, Friedman, and Lin was followed by the benchmark study comprising the combined effort of seven different programs from Europe and North America in which 243 patients were studied retrospectively [1–4]. In 2014 the Food and Drug

P.T. Hoff, M.S., M.D. (✉)
Department of Otolaryngology–Head and Neck Surgery, University of Michigan Health System, Ann Arbor, MI, USA
e-mail: phoff@med.umich.edu

R. Capasso, M.D.
Department of Otolaryngology–Head and Neck Surgery, Sleep Surgery Division, Stanford University Medical Center, Stanford, CA, USA
e-mail: rcapasso@stanford.edu

U. Duvvuri, M.D., Ph.D.
Department of Otolaryngology, University of Pittsburgh, Pittsburgh, PA, USA
e-mail: duvvuriu@upmc.edu

© Springer International Publishing Switzerland 2016

C. Vicini et al. (eds.), *TransOral Robotic Surgery for Obstructive Sleep Apnea*,
DOI 10.1007/978-3-319-34040-1_20

Administration (FDA) approved TORS for removal of benign tissue from the base of tongue, not a complete endorsement of TORS for OSA, but enough to demonstrate safety and efficacy in this setting [5]. To date over 500 TORS cases for OSA have been performed in North America [6].

20.2 The Ann Arbor Experience

The TORS program at St. Joseph Mercy health system (SJMHS) in Ann Arbor, Michigan is the largest single-institution experience in North America with over 220 cases completed since 2010. The setting is a 500-bed community hospital with a robust robotics program encompassing cardiac, thoracic, colorectal, gynecology, urology, and head and neck surgery. At SJMHS over 600 robotic cases were performed in 2014; otolaryngology utilization represented 5 % of total volume, which is fairly representative of most robotics programs.

We began performing TORS for OSA in 2010. Beginning in 2012 the volume of TORS cases for OSA rose sharply; however as we have learned more about predictors of success, patient selection has improved resulting in a dramatic decline in TORS volume and the annual TORS volume has decreased dramatically over compared to the peak years 2012–2013 (Fig. 20.1). As the volume of TORS cases has decreased, the volume of non-TORS multilevel surgery has increased, particularly the use of hyoid myotomy and thyrohoidpexy for cases where DISE demonstrates retrolingual collapse without lymphoid hyperplasia and or secondary epiglottic prolapse. The further addition of the Inspire® hypoglossal nerve stimulator is another tool for retrolingual collapse that may affect TORS volume.

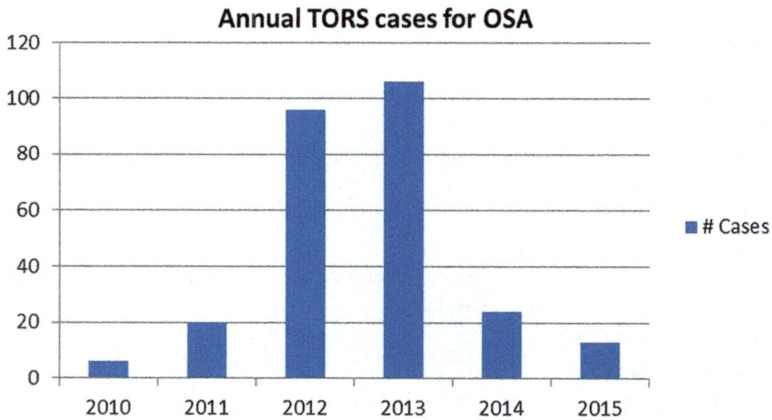

Fig. 20.1 TORS cases for OSA (2015 represents cases performed through July 2015)

20.2.1 *How to Get Started in TORS*

Identify a colleague with similar interest in robotic surgery; this collaboration will give you an eager partner as you begin training in robotic surgery. The experience at SJMHS was successful as a result of this model; one surgeon was interested in the application of TORS for OSA and the other, a head and neck surgeon, was interested in the oncologic application of TORS.

Early in your experience it is very helpful to board cases with one partner acting as console surgeon and the other as bedside assistant; both will learn room setup details and more importantly the intricacies of positioning the robot. As experience and confidence grow the bedside assistant may transition from a co-surgeon to a qualified resident, surgical nurse assistant, or physician assistant.

Attend robotics courses as this is a prerequisite to perform TORS. In the past these courses have included a live animal dissection lab at one of the corporate training sites followed by a masters-level cadaver course hosted by experienced transoral robotic surgeons.

Studies have been performed assessing predictors of successful surgeon training and subsequent implementation of TORS programs [6]. The number of cases performed in the first months after training is predictive of the future success of the program. It is helpful to batch cases so that learned experience can be quickly applied: two cases per day for the novice increasing to four cases per day as experience grows (20–40 cases to become expert). Most successful high-volume programs perform between 25 and 50 cases annually.

Engage colleagues in sleep medicine as they will be your most important source of referrals. Volunteer to participate in or develop an alternative to sleep apnea clinic. This can be a virtual clinic or a formal clinic and should be followed by a formal presentation and discussion of patients to a board comprised of representatives from sleep medicine, otolaryngology, oral surgery, and sleep dentistry; representatives from nutrition and bariatric surgery can also be involved. Give informational talks to referring physician in internal medicine, family medicine, neurology, cardiology, and others. Also consider speaking at American Sleep Apnea Association AWAKE network meetings. Become the sleep surgery expert in your region.

Surgeons incorporating TORS as part of a multilevel treatment of OSA should be very selective when identifying patients for surgery. TORS for OSA is still in its infancy and much work has yet to be done in predicting surgical success and failure. Follow the known predictors of success as you start out:

1. Perform DISE on all patients being considered for sleep surgery of any kind
   (a) Unfavorable findings on DISE suggesting poor surgical outcome:
      - Concentric collapse in the velum, oropharynx, or hypopharynx (tongue)
      - High muscular tongue
      - Small lingual tonsils (Friedman 0–2)
      - Prior pharyngeal surgery for OSA [7]

(b) Findings on DISE suggesting favorable surgical outcome:
   - Large, low lingual tonsils (Friedman 3–4)
   - AP collapse in velum and hypopharynx (tongue)
   - Lateral collapse in oropharynx with palatine tonsils present

2. BMI <30 [8]
3. Friedman stages 2 and 3 [9]
4. Large lingual tonsil volume (surgical volume 7–20 ml)
5. Class 1 or 3 occlusion (avoid class 2)

20.2.2 OR Concerns

20.2.2.1 Robot Block Time

It is critical to establish robot block time and to coordinate this with a designated robot-oriented team; talk with the OR administration and secure TORS block time. TORS for OSA can be performed with any of the da Vinci® platforms, but is probably best done with the Si system® using the 5 mm endo-wrist instruments (Intuitive Surgical®), specifically the Maryland dissector and monopolar cautery spatula.

20.2.2.2 Surgical Team

In addition to robot access, a dedicated surgical technologist and or nurse dedicated to lead a TORS team is critical to the success of the program. The team will increase efficiency and reduce OR turnover time (under 30 min at SJMHC).

20.2.2.3 DISE

This can be a surprising hurdle. Equipment needs are minimal, but are not standard in all operating rooms including:

1. BIS monitoring (Covidien®)
2. Fiber-optic nasopharyngoscope/pediatric bronchoscope
3. Video and audio recording capability

Schedule sleep endoscopy on patients under consideration for TORS. Establish a sedation protocol that is acceptable to both the surgeon and the anesthetist. There is a fair amount of education necessary for the anesthesia team to keep this consistent. Target-controlled infusion (TCI), which is widely used in Europe, is not available in the USA. The University of Pennsylvania has developed a standard protocol for the infusion of Propofol® based on BMI [10]. We and others use manual bolus or constant infusion of Propofol targeting BIS level between 60 and 70 to correspond with fiber-optic observations of the airway.

20.2.3 Credentialing

Every hospital will have its own unique robotic surgery credentialing requirements to obtain privileges. Most hospitals will have developed robotic surgery requirements for their urologists and Ob/Gyn surgeon. Typically, hospitals require surgeons to fulfill three proctored cases before granting privileges. Proctors can be identified by the individual home institution or the manufacturer. Once privileges are obtained many hospitals will require demonstration of continued proficiency. In Ann Arbor robotic surgeons are required to perform 12 cases per year in order to maintain certification. It is recommended that the novice surgeon visit other institutions to learn from experienced colleagues through case observations.

20.2.4 Research

TORS surgeons are at the forefront of head and neck surgery. All surgeons who are beginning a TORS program for OSA, or those who have already adopted TORS into their surgical armamentarium, should consider engaging in clinical research as there is much to learn about the efficacy of this and other techniques for the treatment of OSA. The International Sleep Surgery Society (ISSS) is an excellent venue specifically focused on the surgical treatment of sleep apnea and offers opportunities for collaborative research. ISSS is currently enrolling patients in the international sleep cohort registry (ISCORE), a prospective study evaluating the efficacy of multilevel surgery in patients with moderate-to-severe OSA.

20.2.5 Marketing

Marketing is an important component of building a TORS practice. It is imperative that one develop a working relationship with regional sleep labs and sleep physicians as these will be the greatest source of referrals.

As experience and confidence grow there is an opportunity to explore television, radio, and print marketing. Mailings to referring practices to introduce TORS as a viable new option for patients with OSA can be helpful. Direct marketing to patients is very effective, but can be expensive and is best developed as part of a hospital's comprehensive robotics program; this can include television advertisements and infomercials. Patients utilize the Internet as a first source of information; therefore it is important to develop a website describing OSA treatment options and the surgeon's qualifications. Patient testimonials are very helpful and should be included in the website and in other marketing campaigns.

20.3 University of Pittsburgh Experience

It is now well recognized that OSA is a multilevel disease, with the sites of obstruction ranging from the nasal cavity to the tracheal inlet. TORS has been used to treat obstructive anatomy from the soft palate to the hypopharyngeal area. At the University of Pittsburgh, we have opted to concentrate the use of TORS to only treat the tongue base/retrolingual region.

The modality of treatment is driven by the patient symptoms and, most importantly, the physical examination. The decision-making algorithm has been described above and includes the use of DISE and awake flexible laryngoscopy. On the basis of these investigations, we make a determination about the anatomic site that is responsible for the greater obstruction. This region is then addressed preferentially. That is, if the nasal examination demonstrates significant obstruction, we recommend that the patient undergo a septoplasty as the initial operation. The patient is then evaluated after healing is completed to determine if the retrolingual area still requires surgical correction. We prefer to perform TORS surgery for the tongue base as a single-stage operation. This avoids the risk of circumferential stricture of the oropharynx if tonsillectomy and/or pharyngoplasty are performed at the same time.

With appropriate patient selection, we have seen good success using TORS tongue base resection to reduce both AHI and subjective patient symptoms. Additionally, these results can be augmented if the patients adhere to a weight loss regimen as well. Most realistically, we educate patients with high AHI scores and/or severe symptoms that the surgery is likely to improve their symptoms and result in reducing CPAP pressure settings.

20.4 Stanford Experience

Stanford is one of the pioneering centers in the surgical management of OSA. We have three surgeons with full academic and clinical focus to the field, as well as highly competitive surgical fellowship, medical sleep fellowship program, and opportunity for research positions every year. We aim to provide comprehensive management of snoring and sleep apnea.

Specifically, to address the hypopharyngeal obstruction, we may select patients to undergo either TORS, hypoglossal nerve stimulation implant, radiofrequency ablation of the tongue and tongue base, midline glossectomy, or skeletal surgery.

We have had very promising initial results with the use of TORS, and in general, we encourage patients to consider TORS of the tongue base as one of their possible treatment options. Patients with additional findings of epiglottic collapse on DISE may be candidates to undergo robotic epiglottopexy (suturing of the apex of the epiglottis to tongue base) or partial epiglottectomy.

Although TORS is an efficient technology for access and visualization to the tongue base and epiglottis, we have found that surgery is notable for a particular set of postoperative side effects, especially increased pain, swelling, temporary dysphagia, and tongue paresthesia in comparison to other modalities (e.g., radiofrequency ablations, and hypoglossal nerve stimulator). As such, besides taking into consideration the clinical presentation, physical examination, craniofacial anatomy, sleep study, and in some cases drug-induced sleep endoscopy (DISE) and/or radiologic findings, we actively involve the patients in the decision to proceed with the treatment paradigm. We spend a significant amount of time counseling the patients preoperatively so that they are well educated as to the role, rationale, risks, and alternatives of TORS for sleep apnea.

In addition, whereas TORS is an exciting innovation to the field of surgery, cost-effectiveness issues in applications for sleep surgery do remain a significant concern at this time. Third-party payers have yet to fully recognize the added value of this technology in the treatment of snoring and sleep apnea. The length of time and cost required for the surgery may be increased as compared to traditional techniques. Expected advances in the technology will make this technology prove even more useful.

20.5 Conclusion

Developing a TORS program in North America is only limited by the surgeon's interest in committing to collaboration with sleep specialists in his or her community and a commitment by the institution to provided adequate robot block time to make the program viable. Robotic surgery has been popular in the USA since its widespread application in urologic surgery. Many surgical specialties including cardiac, thoracic, colorectal, gynecology, urology, and head and neck surgeons compete for the robot. In the USA most hospitals have one or more da Vinci robots. However, our colleagues in Canada are not so fortunate and therefore have not offered TORS as part of their treatment of OSA.

The instrumentation needs for TORS are minimal, as are the equipment needs for DISE. A dedicated TORS surgical team will optimize efficiencies in the operating room and will allow the surgeon to utilize a nurse or surgical nurse to act as the bedside assistant. Most surgeons perform DISE either as a stand-alone procedure or at the time of planned multilevel surgery. The use of TCI is not available in the USA, but alternative methods have been developed [10]. The comfort level anesthesiologists have with DISE will vary, but with education and patience, this obstacle can be easily overcome. Marketing is an important tool, but should be used judiciously when first starting out.

Finally, TORS for OSA is in its infancy and all surgeons performing this procedure as part of a multilevel treatment of OSA should create a database and endeavor to share their results either individually or by collaborative efforts through the ISSS.

References

1. Vicini C, Dallan I, Canzi P, Frassineti S, La Pietra MG, Montevecchi F. Transoral robotic tongue base resection in obstructive sleep apnoea-hypopnoea syndrome: a preliminary report. ORL J Otorhinolaryngol Relat Spec. 2010;72(1):22–7.
2. Lin HS, Rowley JA, Badr MS, Folbe AJ, Yoo GH, Victor L, Mathog RH, Chen W. Transoral robotic surgery for treatment of obstructive sleep apnea-hypopnea syndrome. Laryngoscope. 2013;123(7):1811–6. doi:10.1002/lary.23913.
3. Friedman M, Hamilton C, Samuelson CG, Kelley K, Taylor D, Pearson-Chauhan K, Maley A, Taylor R, Venkatesan TK. Transoral robotic glossectomy for the treatment of obstructive sleep apnea-hypopnea syndrome. Otolaryngol Head Neck Surg. 2012;146(5):854–62.
4. Vicini C, Montevecchi F, Campanini A, Dallan I, Hoff PT, Spector ME, Thaler E, Ahn J, Baptista P, Remacle M, Lawson G, Benazzo M, Canzi P. Clinical outcomes and complications associated with TORS for OSAHS: a benchmark for evaluating an emerging surgical technology in a targeted application for benign disease. ORL J Otorhinolaryngol Relat Spec. 2014;76(2):63–9.
5. Hoff PT, D'Agostino MA, Thaler ER. Transoral robotic surgery in benign diseases including obstructive sleep apnea: safety and feasibility. Laryngoscope. 2015;125(5):1249–53.
6. Intuitive data: frequency of TORS after training and successful implementation of TORS.
7. Thaler ER, Rassekh CH, Lee JM, Weinstein GS, O'Malley Jr BW. Outcomes for multilevel surgery for sleep apnea: obstructive sleep apnea, transoral robotic surgery, and uvulopalatopharyngoplasty. Laryngoscope. 2016;126(1):266–9.
8. Hoff PT, Glazer TA, Spector ME. Body mass index predicts success in patients undergoing transoral robotic surgery for obstructive sleep apnea. ORL J Otorhinolaryngol Relat Spec. 2014;76(5):266–72.
9. Spector M, Glazer T, Hoff P. Multilevel surgery for obstructive sleep apnea with TORS base of tongue reduction: outcomes stratified by Friedman stage. ORL 2016;78(1):1–8.
10. Atkins JH, Mandel JE, Rosanova G. Safety and efficacy of drug-induced sleep endoscopy using a probability ramp propofol infusion system in patients with severe obstructive sleep apnea. Anesth Analg. 2014;119(4):805–10.

Chapter 21
The South American Experience

Eric R. Thuler, Fábio A.W. Rabelo, and Fabiana C.P. Valera

21.1 Introduction

The technology of da Vinci robotic surgery is still not a reality for the great majority of hospitals in Latin America. In 2015, there are only 44 Da Vinci platforms for robotic surgery (Intuitive®) in Latin America (out of approximately 3102 robotic platforms worldwide). According to Intuitive, this technology is available in ten countries (Brazil, Mexico, Argentina, Chile, Colombia, Venezuela, Ecuador, Uruguay, Panama and Dominican Republic) and most of them are available mainly for urologists, general surgeons and gynecologists. Very few centers rely on otorhinolaryngologists certified for da Vinci use.

21.2 The Brazilian Experience

In Brazil, the Da Vinci Platform is available mainly in private hospitals, out of 14 hospitals only two are public. Although the researches are more concentrated in public health system and they could facilitate propagation of these new technologies, the relatively high cost of Da Vinci associated to elevated taxes make this

E.R. Thuler, M.D.
Robotic Surgery Center at Oswaldo Cruz German Hospital, São Paulo, Brazil

Department of ICEP, Hospital Sirio-Libanês, São Paulo, Brazil

F.A.W. Rabelo, M.D., Ph.D. (✉)
Robotic Surgery Center at Oswaldo Cruz German Hospital, São Paulo, Brazil
e-mail: fawrabelo@hotmail.com

F.C.P. Valera, M.D., Ph.D.
Department of Ophthalmology, Otorhinolaryngology and Head and Neck Surgery, ENT Division, Medical School of Ribeirão Preto, University of São Paulo, Ribeirão Preto, Brazil

© Springer International Publishing Switzerland 2016

C. Vicini et al. (eds.), *TransOral Robotic Surgery for Obstructive Sleep Apnea*,
DOI 10.1007/978-3-319-34040-1_21

technology unfeasible for most hospitals, especially the public ones. For this reason, TORS and other robotic surgeries are available for a very limited number of persons. The first center to acquire the system from Intuitive was Albert Einstein Jewish Hospital in 2008. The first TORS procedure was performed for cancer in Syrian-Lebanese Hospital in 2010.

Until the early twentieth century, surgical treatment for Obstructive Sleep Apnea Syndrome (OSAS) basically was represented by pharyngeal surgeries like uvulopalatopharyngoplasty (UPPP), but results with these techniques were very inconsistent [1–3]. For us, the need to approach the tongue base was especially observed since the initial research with Drug Induced Sleep Endoscopy, at the School of Medicine of Ribeirão Preto—University of São Paulo, in 2005 [4, 5]. The research in DISE started to improve patient selection for UPPP and the surgical results, but since the first DISE cases the hypopharyngeal collapse took our attention [6] due to its frequency, and to the relationship of its presence to UPPP surgical failure [7, 8].

Since 2010, we have extended DISE indication for all patients with failure in CPAP adherence. Hypopharyngeal collapse corresponded to about 40 % of the obstructive sites: the lingual tonsil hypertrophy and the epiglottis were involved in almost 15 % of the cases [9], motivating the search for a solution for these cases.

By this time, the contact with Prof. Vicini and his team, one of the most experienced groups in TORS for OSAS [10], was essential. We could visit Forli Hospital several times, and we could follow their routine and find out the feasibility and safety of robotic surgery. The contact with Prof. Vicini and the Da Vinci Platform motivated us to find a way to bring this procedure to Brazil.

After been properly certificated, we (ET + FR) performed our first five cases with Prof. Vicini in Syrian-Lebanese Hospital in 2013, since then we have performed 20 cases of TORS for OSAS, five cases with surgery only in tongue base and epiglottis and 12 associated with expansion pharyngoplasty. Our results are in process to be published, the average age is 37 years (±7,6), BMI 27 (±3,4), preoperative AHI 23,6 (±5,7) and postoperative AHI 5,3 (±3,6). We had two failures, with a success rate of 90 %.

Even though the technique first described includes tracheostomy for the procedure, we chose to perform them with nasal intubation. This choice was due to some new studies that gave support for performing without tracheostomy [11, 12] and because the patients were younger and with low BMI. Besides that the acceptance of surgery here would be higher without the tracheostomy.

Currently our group is the only one that currently performs TORS for OSAS in two private hospitals: Syrian-Lebanese Hospital and Oswaldo Cruz German Hospital, both in São Paulo. The last one has recently created the first robotic center focusing also in OSAS treatment.

Our next step is to collaborate, disseminate and expand the use of the robotic system in Latin America, through courses and training programs and also demonstrate and publish appropriate criteria for patient selection for best benefit from this technology.

It is important to mention that Chile and Argentina are developing good programs in Robotic Surgery and surgeons are starting to direct TORS for OSAS. Colombia is another country with an important robotic surgery center that did the first TORS case for OSAS last year (2014).

In general, robotic surgery technology is currently cost prohibitive resulting in limited access particularly in Latin American countries where limited resources for health care is common. However, over time, costs will decrease and technology will become more accessible. Assuming this, it is important to propagate the use of the da Vinci or similar robotic platforms, showing advantages and disadvantages, demonstrating that when properly indicated the results are good and the robotic system is a promising tool.

References

1. Aurora RN, Casey KR, Kristo D, Auerbach S, Bista SR, Chowdhuri S, Karippot A, Lamm C, Ramar K, Zak R, Morgenthaler TI. Practice parameters for the surgical modifications of the upper airway for obstructive sleep apnea in adults. Sleep. 2010;33(10):1408–13.
2. Caples SM, Rowley JA, Prinsell JR, Pallanch JF, Elamin MB, Katz SG, Harwick JD. Surgical modifications of the upper airway for obstructive sleep apnea in adults: a systematic review and meta-analysis. Sleep. 2010;33(10):1396–407.
3. Sundaram S, Bridgman SA, Lim J, Lasserson TJ. Surgery for obstructive sleep apnoea/hypopnoea syndrome. Cochrane Database Syst Rev. 2005;4:CD001004. Review.
4. Rabelo FA, Braga A, Küpper DS, De Oliveira JA, Lopes FM, de Lima Mattos PL, Barreto SG, Sander HH, Fernandes RM, Valera FC. Propofol-induced sleep: polysomnographic evaluation of patients with obstructive sleep apnea and controls. Otolaryngol Head Neck Surg. 2010;142(2):218–24.
5. Rabelo FA, Küpper DS, Sander HH, Fernandes RM, Valera FC. Polysomnographic evaluation of propofol-induced sleep in patients with respiratory sleep disorders and controls. Laryngoscope. 2013;123(9):2300–5.
6. Campanini A, Canzi P, De Vito A, Dallan I, Montevecchi F, Vicini C. Awake versus sleep endoscopy: personal experience in 250 OSAHS patients. Acta Otorhinolaryngol Ital. 2010;30(2):73–7.
7. Koutsourelakis I, Saffirudin F, Ravesloot M, Zakynthinos S. Surgery for obstructive sleep apnea : sleep endoscopy determinants of outcome. Laryngoscope. 2012;122(11):2587–91.
8. Kezirian EJ. Nonresponders to pharyngeal surgery for obstructive sleep apnea: insights from drug-induced sleep endoscopy. Laryngoscope. 2011;121(6):1320–6.
9. Rabelo FAW, Küpper DS, Haueisen Sander H, dos Santos V, Thuler E, França Fernandes RM, et al. A comparison of the Fujita classification of awake and drug-induced sleep endoscopy patients. Braz J Otorhinolaryngol. 2013;79(1):100–5.
10. Vicini C, Montevecchi F, Campanini A, Dallan I, Hoff PT, Spector ME, et al. Clinical outcomes and complications associated with TORS for OSAHS: a benchmark for evaluating an emerging surgical technology in a targeted application for benign disease. ORL J Otorhinolaryngol Relat Spec. 2014;76(2):63–9.
11. Lin H, Rowley JA, Badr MS, Folbe AJ, Yoo GH, Victor L, et al. Transoral robotic surgery for treatment of obstructive sleep apnea-hypopnea syndrome. Laryngoscope. 2015;125(4):1013–20.
12. Hoffmann TK, Schuler PJ, Bankfalvi A, Greve J, Heusgen L, Lang S, et al. Comparative analysis of resection tools suited for transoral robot-assisted surgery. Eur Arch Otorhinolaryngol. 2013;271(5):1207–13.

Chapter 22
The European Experience

Asit Arora, Bhik Kotecha, Tom Vauterin, Guillermo Plaza, Christian Güldner, and Jochen A. Werner

22.1 Introduction

Vicini et al. first performed TORS for OSAH in Italy in 2008, as a modification of open tongue base reduction and hyoid epiglottopexy [1]. Since this time, several other units across Europe have established similar TORS programs to treat this condition. The following section provides an overview of the experience of four such programs from the UK, Belgium, Spain and Germany.

A. Arora, Ph.D., D.I.C., F.R.C.S. (✉)
Department of Otorhinolaryngology and Head & Neck Surgery, St. Mary's Hospital, Imperial College Healthcare NHS Trust, London, UK
e-mail: asitarora@doctors.org.uk

B. Kotecha, M.B.B.Ch., M.Phil., F.R.C.S.
Royal National Throat Nose and Ear Hospital, London, UK

T. Vauterin, M.D.
Department of Otorhinolaryngology, Head and Neck Surgery, AZ Sint-Jan Bruges-Ostend, Brugge, Belgium
e-mail: tom.vauterin@azsintjan.be

G. Plaza, M.D., Ph.D.
Hospital Universitario de Fuenlabrada and Hospital Sanitas La Zarzuela, Fuenlabrada, Spain
e-mail: gplaza.hflr@salud.madrid.org

C. Güldner, M.D., Ph.D. • J.A. Werner, M.D.
University Hospital of Essen, Essen, Germany
e-mail: gueldner@staff.uni-marburg.de; jochen.werner@uk-essen.de

© Springer International Publishing Switzerland 2016

C. Vicini et al. (eds.), *TransOral Robotic Surgery for Obstructive Sleep Apnea*,
DOI 10.1007/978-3-319-34040-1_22

22.2 The UK Experience

22.2.1 Background

In the UK, the first robotic program in ENT was established at St. Mary's Hospital, Imperial College London, by Mr. Neil Tolley and Mr. Asit Arora in 2009. A subsequent collaboration with Mr. Bhik Kotecha at the Royal National Throat Nose and Ear Hospital, London, was established in 2010 to apply TORS for treating patients with OSA who have failed conventional treatment modalities. This team has performed approximately 40 cases to date, carefully selecting patients using drug-induced sedation endoscopy (DISE) to identify potential candidates for TORS. Patients are eligible for treatment within the public (National Healthcare Service) system. Clinical evaluation is conducted within the context of a national ethically approved prospective study.

To date, there are 44 hospitals in the UK with a da Vinci system. In the last 3 years, six other ENT departments have established a robotic program although only one of these, in Newcastle, is also using TORS for patients with sleep-disordered breathing. As is the case in other countries, notably Belgium, there is the potential for many more departments to start a TORS program for OSAS given the number of hospitals in the UK with a da Vinci system. Nevertheless, as evident in Spain, access to the da Vinci is often restricted by its use in other specialties, particularly urology.

22.2.2 Guidelines and Patient Selection

To date there are no formal UK guidelines available. TORS is generally reserved as a 'final option' when all other existing treatment options have failed. Criteria for offering TORS for OSAH within the context of NHS healthcare provision include patients with (1) moderate-to-severe OSA confirmed by sleep study (defined as an apnoea-hypopnoea index (AHI) ≥15 episodes/h); (2) failure or refusal of all other treatment modalities including CPAP, mandibular advancement device (MAD), and surgery; (3) BMI less than 35 kg/cm^2 and (4) predominant BOT collapse with or without epiglottic collapse evaluated by DISE. All patients undergo robotic-assisted tongue base reduction (TBR) and those with concurrent epiglottic prolapse identified by DISE, also undergo wedge epiglottoplasty. The possibility of intensive care admission, nasogastric tube insertion and tracheostomy is routinely included as part of the standard consent process.

22.2.3 Technique

Nasotracheal intubation is performed to facilitate access to the tongue base and epiglottis. The operating room configuration described by O'Malley et al. is used [2]. Tongue base reduction is performed by thulium laser ablation (2013 nm, 15 W), commencing in the midline from the foramen caecum and circumvallate papillae to the vallecula. A 1 cm mucosal bridge between the base of the epiglottis and the tongue represents the posterior limit and is employed to minimise oedema at the epiglottic base. The lateral limits are 1 cm to either side of the midline to a depth of 2 cm. Any excess lingual tonsillar tissue is additionally ablated down to muscle. Regarding epiglottic resection, a wedge-shaped laser excision of the upper one-half of the epiglottis is performed. The plane of resection is above the pharyngo-epiglottic folds to minimise the chance of aspiration and to avoid bleeding from branches of the superior laryngeal artery.

22.2.4 Peri-operative Management

All patients receive perioperative and post-operative steroids (dexamethasone 2 mg three times daily for 5 days) to minimise swelling, nausea and pain. In addition, antibiotics are given (co-amoxiclav 625 mg three times daily for 5 days), analgesia (paracetamol 1 g four times daily, ibuprofen 400 mg three times daily, and codeine 30 mg as required) and benzydamine hydrochloride gargles (4–6 times daily for 2 weeks). Usually patients are discharged within 24 h after surgery having been commenced on a soft diet. Nasogastric tube insertion and tracheostomy have not been required in any of the patients to date.

22.2.5 Outcome

The preliminary results are encouraging and a 64 % cure rate has been achieved with a normal post-operative sleep study in 36 % of cases. No major complications have been witnessed. Minor bleeding which settled with conservative measures was a complication observed in one patient. The vast majority of patients start a soft diet immediately after surgery and swallow function returns to normal after 4 weeks. A sustained reduction in the mean Epworth Sleep Score and significant improvement in quality of life measures were evident 24 months following surgery [3].

22.2.6 *Other Considerations*

The TORS technique utilised in the UK can be but is usually not part of extensive multilevel surgery as reported in the literature by most other units. The laser ablation technique used for tongue base reduction may represent a less aggressive technique compared with resection. In accordance with others, TORS for BOT reduction can be safely performed without the need for tracheostomy or conversion to open surgery [4, 5]. A success rate of 64 % was achieved based on Sher criteria [6]. This is consistent with other studies that report success rates of 45–90 % with TORS [4, 7–10].

22.3 The Belgian Experience

22.3.1 *Background*

In Belgium over 30 hospitals currently use the da Vinci system for urological and gynecological procedures. Since the approval of TORS by the FDA in 2009, approximately ten ENT departments established a robotic program. Of these, four use TORS for sleep-disordered breathing: AZ Sint-Jan Hospital Bruges—Ostend, University Hospital Antwerp, AZ Sint-Lucas Hospital Ghent and University Hospital Namur. Considering the number of robotic systems in Belgium, there is a high potential for ENT departments to start a TORS programme for OSAS in the future.

22.3.2 *Guidelines and Patient Selection*

To date there are no Belgian guidelines available. On a European level, the European Respiratory Society (ERS) task force report concerning non-CPAP therapies for OSAS does not mention TORS [11]. TORS should be seen as another way of performing conventional procedures of the oropharynx. Therefore, guidelines of these conventional procedures should apply to robotic procedures, but possibly with better outcome.

The main indication for TORS in sleep-disordered breathing is OSAS. We consider TORS in an OSAS patient when CPAP is not tolerated or wanted by the patient, or when CPAP is not reimbursed (apnoea hypopnoea index (AHI) of less than 20 per hour). Occasionally, TORS is used in patients with isolated snoring. In such cases, these patients need to be strongly motivated.

Surgery is performed in centres where there is a specific multidisciplinary programme for OSAS and snoring. Patient evaluation is always performed in close collaboration with colleagues from respiratory medicine, maxillofacial surgery and neurology and consists of clinical examination, laryngoscopy and polysomnography.

When surgery is considered DISE is performed to select patients for the most appropriate surgical procedure. Tongue base collapse should be observed on DISE prior to consideration of TORS-assisted tongue base reduction. Belgian centres consider TORS as a better alternative to perform tongue base reduction than laser surgery.

If necessary, an additional simultaneous procedure to address the soft palate and lateral pharynx may be indicated and selected accordingly.

Mandibular advancement treatments (with osteotomies or a device) are recognised as a valuable alternative.

Finally, patients are informed about the additional cost of TORS. If this is a financial problem for the patient, trans-oral laser surgery (TLS) is an option, although we believe that this is a less optimal operative technique.

22.3.3 Technique

As with other surgical procedures, it is difficult to describe a uniform technique for different centres. Most hospitals use the da Vinci Si system, and some the MedRobotics-Flex-System. Some centres only do isolated robotic tongue base procedures whilst others combine this with conventional oropharyngeal surgery. Some always perform epiglottoplasty when reducing the tongue base whilst others only do so when circular collapse of the epiglottis is witnessed at DISE. As is the case in the UK and Spain, tracheostomy is not routinely performed in TORS. In our centre we use the 30° endoscope, the Maryland bipolar forceps and the unipolar cautery installed at the three robotic arms.

22.3.4 Other Considerations

Because of the strict selection criteria, TORS for sleep-disordered breathing is not a common procedure. Approximately 90 robotic sleep-disordered breathing procedures were performed in Belgium in the last 5 years. In this way we feel that it is important to perform TORS for head and neck cancer and chronic lingual tonsillar hypertrophy to improve expertise and to shorten the learning curve.

22.4 The Spanish Experience

22.4.1 Background

As in many other countries in Europe, treatment of oropharyngeal pathology has been performed using trans-oral laser microsurgery (TLM) in recent years. Thus, the introduction of TORS to treat such cases has been delayed to some extent by this practice and the TLM expertise evident across the country.

In 2011, the first TORS case was performed in Pamplona, in 2011, after Dr. Peter Baptista had been trained in TORS. Although the da Vinci system is available throughout many hospitals in Spain, TORS as a treatment for OSA is only performed in a few selected centres. This includes two private hospitals (Clínica Universitaria de Navarra, Pamplona, and Hospital Sanitas La Zarzuela, Madrid) and a public hospital (Hospital Rey Juan Carlos, Móstoles, Madrid). Just recently, two more hospitals in Madrid have acquired a da Vinci robot and may start a TORS programme. Specifically, at Hospital Quiron (Madrid), Prof. Julio Acero, a maxillofacial surgeon, has been recently trained in TORS. In contrast, the public system of hospitals does not promote any TORS program, although there are several robots available.

22.4.2 Guidelines and Patient Selection

In Spain there are national guidelines for OSA diagnosis and treatment. However, this does not include tongue base surgery of any kind. Therefore, for every patient, the correct indication must be established through a complete physical exam and significant findings during DISE. The latter is in accordance with the DISE protocol established to diagnose and manage OSA patients. Thereafter, local OSA committees are key to help to find the right candidates. Potential candidates for TORS are similar to those in the UK, namely patients with OSA when the AHI is >25 and CPAP is not tolerated.

22.4.3 Technique

In contrast to UK practice, surgery is usually performed in a multilevel fashion, with pharyngoplasty and/or septoplasty also performed as indicated. The da Vinci Si system is currently used to perform tongue base reduction and epiglottoplasty and in keeping with other European centres, tracheostomy is not routinely performed [6, 8, 11–13].

In total, we have performed TORS in approximately 70 cases of OSA across three hospitals in Spain over the last 4 years. The team at Pamplona has performed 43 cases, 16 cases have been performed at Hospital Sanitas La Zarzuela and in Móstoles, in the public system, three TORS cases have been performed for OSA. It is noticeable that in the private hospital setting it is easier to establish and perform a programme of TORS for OSA compared to the public sector. This is because in the latter, use of the robot is more restricted in non-oncological cases.

22.4.4 *Outcome*

Different authors have reported success in most cases. Our results are similar, with AHI reductions by half in more than 80 % patients, when TORS has been correctly indicated and performed. Nevertheless, complications are an important issue [14]. Bleeding after the procedure has been a major problem in three cases (out of 70) with one patient requiring an emergency tracheostomy. Pain and severe dysphagia lasting as long as 3 weeks are common and patients should be appropriately consented [15].

22.4.5 *Other Considerations*

Establishing a TORS programme is associated with numerous challenges. Once the robot is available in any hospital in Spain, it usually 'belongs' to the urologic department, which is able to easily perform 50–75 cases per year. It is very important to discuss the need to use the robot for TORS with the local managers so that we are 'allowed' to use this equipment on a regular basis. When using the laser, usually it is to the contrary: this equipment traditionally 'belongs' to the ENT department.

Cost is also an important issue. Our health system does not cover the additional costs that TORS require. Once TORS has been proposed to a patient, it is the responsibility of their local ENT team to search for the necessary financial support to make surgery possible. This is difficult in the public setting and very demanding for the patient in the private sector.

Going forward, patient selection for TORS needs to be optimised. DISE is a mandatory tool in this regard [16]. MRI may also provide important additional information to determine how much tissue needs to be removed during TORS and to establish the exact location of lingual arteries and branches to avoid unnecessary damage and bleeding [16].

Furthermore, the TORS technique should also be improved. Maryland forceps were not designed for TORS and better grasping forceps are needed. Decreasing the optic size and increasing the flexibility of surgical instruments would also be beneficial.

22.5 The German Experience

22.5.1 *Background*

In general, trans-oral surgery has been practiced in Germany for many decades, mostly in the form of trans-oral laser surgery (TLS). Consequently, TLS is established as a standard therapy for benign and malignant disease, as well as in OSAS surgery [18–21]. Therefore, as is the situation in Spain, TORS has had to 'compete' with TLS. Comparative studies have not been published, so the benefit of TORS over TLS is not proven. In our own experience, TLS has a broad spectrum of indications and regarding patient outcome TORS seems to be at least as good as TLM in selected patient groups.

Following FDA approval of TORS in 2009, ENT departments across the country began to adopt this technique. At the present time, nine centres (out of 38 university hospitals and an additional 120 ENT departments) have an established robotic programme. These are the University Hospital Heidelberg (2010); University Hospital Essen (2011); University Hospital Hamburg (2011); Prosper Hospital Recklinghausen (2011); University Hospital Erlangen (2012); University Hospital Marburg (2012); University Hospital Homburg (2012); St. Elizabeth Hospital Straubing (2012) and University Hospital Ulm (2013). Approximately 20 additional otolaryngology departments have the potential to start a TORS programme due to the fact that there is a da Vinci system available in their hospital.

22.5.2 Guidelines and Patient Selection

Regarding the use of TORS in OSAS surgery, TORS has not been included in German guidelines of operative therapy for OSAS or snoring thus far [22, 23].

22.5.3 Technique

In our opinion TORS simply represents another technique to perform an operation, so strategies like reduction of base of tongue or UVPP can be performed by TORS as well as by conventional operation techniques. Consequently, in Marburg, we performed ten operations with focus on surgical OSAS therapy using two robotic systems: the da Vinci and the MedRobotics-Flex-System.

22.5.4 Outcome

The advantage of TORS in comparison with TLS was the improvement of visualisation, especially in base of tongue due to the 30°-angled optic system. Other German centres report similar experiences in personal discussion.

22.5.5 *Other Considerations*

The delayed adoption of TORS is at least in part due to the differences in health-care structure in Germany compared to the USA. In Germany, the health system is based on diagnose-related-group-system (DRG) where insurance providers do not cover the additional costs which are about 800–1000€ per case [4–23].

Another factor related to poor adoption is the issue concerning the reprocessing of used instruments and the need for different cleaning techniques for robotic equipment. This has led to the establishment of a completely new set of procedures of reprocessing, i.e. cleaning, disinfection and sterilisation, which have to be altered and adapted to the German regulations of the Commission for Hospital Hygiene and Infection Prevention at the Robert Koch Institute (RKI), the Federal Institute for Drugs and Medical Devices (BfArM) and the DIN EN ISO 17664 [24].

22.6 Summary

TORS for OSA is only established in a few selected centres in the UK, Germany, Spain and Belgium. There are no consensus national guidelines for TORS and OSA and as a result TORS is only being used for sleep-disordered breathing in a fraction of centres. Careful patient selection on a case-by-case basis and in a multidisciplinary setting is important. In all the European centres reported, TORS represents a new treatment paradigm for OSA patients that do not tolerate CPAP. DISE is universally used to guide patient selection and the surgical technique is particularly useful to treat tongue base hypertrophy and epiglottic prolapse.

References

1. Vicini C, Dallan I, Canzi P, Frassineti S, La Pietra MG, Montevecchi F. Transoral robotic tonge base resection in obstructive sleep apnoea-hypopnoea syndrome: a preliminary report. ORL J Otorhinolaryngol Relat Spec. 2010;72(1):22–7.
2. O'Malley Jr BW, Weinstein GS, Snyder W, Hockstein NG. Transoral robotic surgery (TORS) for base of tongue neoplasms. Laryngoscope. 2006;116:1465–72.
3. Arora A, Tolley N, Kotecha B, et al. Functional outcomes after Transoral robotic surgery for obstructive sleep apnoea. Clin Otol. 2012;37(S1):97.
4. Friedman M, Hamilton C, Samuelson CG, Kelley K, Taylor D, Pearson-Chauhan K, Maley A, Taylor R, Venkatesan TK. Transoral robotic glossectomy for the treatment of obstructive sleep apnea-hypopnea syndrome. Otolaryngol Head Neck Surg. 2012;146:854–62.
5. Lin HS, Rowley JA, Badr MS, Folbe AJ, Yoo GH, Victor L, Mathoq RH, Chen W. Transoral robotic surgery for treatment of obstructive sleep apnea-hypopnea syndrome. Laryngoscope. 2013;123:1811–6.
6. Arora A, Chaidas K, Garas G, Amlani A, Darzi A, Kotecha B, Tolley NS. Outcome of TORS to tongue base and epiglottis in patients with OSA intolerant of conventional treatment. Sleep Breath. 2015 Dec 15 Ahead of print.

7. Lee JM, Weinstein GS, O'Malley Jr BW, Thaler ER. Transoral robotic-assisted lingual tonsillectomy and uvulopalatopharyngoplasty for obstructive sleep apnea. Ann Otol Rhinol Laryngol. 2012;121:636–9.
8. Vicini C, Montevecchi F, Campanini A, Dallan I, Hoff PT, Spector ME, Thaler E, Ahn J, Baptista P, Remacle M, Lawson G, Benazzo M, Canzi P. Clinical outcomes and complications associated with TORS for OSAHS: a benchmark for evaluating an emerging surgical technology in a targeted application for benign disease. ORL J Otorhinolaryngol Relat Spec. 2014;76:63–9.
9. Toh ST, Han HJ, Tay HN, Kiong KL. Transoral robotic surgery for obstructive sleep apnea in Asian patients: a Singapore sleep centre experience. JAMA Otolaryngol Head Neck Surg. 2014;140:624–9.
10. Randerath WJ, Verbraecken J, Andreas S, Bettega G, Boudewyns A, Hamans E, et al. ERS Task Force Report: non-CPAP therapies in obstructive sleep apnoea. Eur Respir J. 2011;37:1000–28.
11. Vicini C, Montevecchi F, Tenti G, et al. Transoral robotic surgery: tongue base reducction and supraglottoplasty for obstructive sleep apnea. Oper Tech Otolaryngol. 2012;23:45–7.
12. Vicini C, Dallan I, Canzi P, et al. Transoral robotic surgery of the tongue base in obstructive sleep Apnea-Hypopnea syndrome: anatomic considerations and clinical experience. Head Neck. 2012;34:15–22.
13. Vicini C, Montevecchi F, Pang K, et al. Combined transoral robotic tongue base surgery and palate surgery in obstructive sleep apnea-hypopnea syndrome: expansion sphincter pharyngoplasty versus uvulopalatopharyngoplasty. Head Neck. 2014;36:77–83.
14. Hoff PT, D'Agostino MA, Thaler ER. Transoral robotic surgery in benign diseases including obstructive sleep apnea: safety and feasibility. Laryngoscope. 2015;125:1249–53.
15. Eesa M, Montevecchi F, Hendawy E, et al. Swallowing outcome after TORS for sleep apnea: short- and long-term evaluation. Eur Arch Otorhinolaryngol. 2015;272:1537–41.
16. Lin HS, Rowley JA, Folbe AJ, et al. Transoral robotic surgery for treatment of obstructive sleep apnea: factors predicting surgical response. Laryngoscope. 2015;125:1013–20.
17. Chiffer RC, Schwab RJ, Keenan BT, et al. Volumetric MRI analysis pre and post transoral robotic surgery for obstructive sleep apnea (OSA-TORS). Laryngoscope. 2015;125:1988–95.
18. Werner JA. Transoral laser microsurgery in carcinomas of the oral cavity, pharynx, and larynx. Cancer Control. 2002;9(5):379–86.
19. Rudert HH. Endoscopic resections of glottic and supraglottic carcinomas with the CO_2 laser. Eur Arch Otorhinolaryngol. 1995;252(3):146–8.
20. Steiner W. Transoral laser microsurgery for squamous cell carcinoma of the base of the tongue. Arch Otolaryngol Head Neck Surg. 2003;129(1):36–43.
21. Ambrosch P. Carbon dioxide laser microsurgery for early supraglottic carcinoma. Ann Otol Rhinol Laryngol. 1998;107(8):680–8.
22. Verse T. Guideline: treatment of obstructive sleep apnea in adults. HNO. 2009;57(11):1136–56.
23. Stuck BA. Diagnosis and treatment of snoring in adults-S2k Guideline of the German Society of Otorhinolaryngology, Head and Neck Surgery. Sleep Breath. 2015;19(1):135–48.
24. Mandapathil M. Establishing a transoral robotic surgery program in an academic hospital in Germany. Acta Otolaryngol. 2014;134:661–5.

Chapter 23
The Middle East Experience

Medhat Shams and Hayam Altaweel

23.1 Introduction

The epidemic of OSA is closely related to obesity, an important public health related condition facing adults globally. In the USA in 2004, the estimated prevalence of adult obesity, classified as a body mass index (BMI) over 30, was more than 30 %, and the prevalence of extreme obesity (BMI>40) was 2.8 % in men and 6.7 % in women [1].

Qatar is located on a peninsula in the Arab Gulf and its citizens have the highest per capita income in the world. It is also becoming the world's fattest country. With a population of 2.3 million, half of all adults are obese and 17 % of the population suffers from diabetes [2]. Childhood obesity is also a problem with 36.5 % of boys and 23.6 % of girls age 12–17 overweight in 2003. By 2015, it is predicted that 73 % of women and 69 % of men will be obese [3]. According to the International Association for the Study of Obesity, Qatar has the sixth highest rate of obesity among boys in the Middle East and North Africa region. It is also ranked fifth for having the highest percentage of people between 20 and 79 with diabetes.

One reason for the obesity trend is the lack of exercise and poorly designed pedestrian friendly cities. Like other oil-rich nations, Qatar has leaped across decades of development in a short time, leaving behind the physically demanding life of the desert for air-conditioned comfort, servants, and fast food.

Those who are considered overweight have a BMI of 25 or more, while the definition of obesity is with a BMI of 30 or more. Interestingly, although Qatar's population has continued to pile on the pounds, so has much of the rest of the world, putting Qatar now in fifth place globally in terms of its prevalence of overweight

M. Shams, M.D. (✉) • H. Altaweel, F.A.C.H., A.R.Z.T.
Department of Otolaryngology—Head and Neck Surgery, Hamad Medical Corporation, Rumailah Hospital, Doha, Qatar
e-mail: a1shams@hotmail.com; altaweelhayam@yahoo.co.uk

© Springer International Publishing Switzerland 2016
C. Vicini et al. (eds.), *TransOral Robotic Surgery for Obstructive Sleep Apnea*,
DOI 10.1007/978-3-319-34040-1_23

Table 23.1 Overweight and obesity statistics in the Middle East and gulf states

		% of overweight men	% of overweight women	% of obese men	% of obese women	Source	Link to article
Turkey	2001–2002	46.5 %	28.6 %	16.5 %	29. 4 %	8	Obesity in Turkey
Israel	2011	45.8 %	33.1 %	15.4 %	15.9 %	9	Obesity in Israel
Jordan	2002	–	27.6 %	–	26.3 %	8	Obesity in Jordan
Lebanon	1998–2002	–	–	36.3 %	38.3 %	8	Obesity in Lebanon
Palestinian Territories	2003	–	–	23.9%	42.8 %	10	Obesity in Palestine Territories
Bahrain	1998–1999	36.7 %	28.3 %	23.3 %	34.1 %	8	Obesity in Bahrain
Kuwait	1998–2002	36.3 %	32.8 %	27.5 %	29.9 %	8	Obesity in Kuwait
Oman	2000	32.1 %	27.3 %	16.7 %	23.8 %	8	Obesity in Oman
Qatar	2003	34.3 %	33 %	34.6%	45.3 %	8	Obesity in Qatar
Saudi Arabia	1995–2002	42.4 %	31.8 %	26.4 %	44.0 %	8	Obesity in Saudi
United Emirates	2000	36.7 %	28.4 %	17.1 %	31.4 %	8	Obesity in Emirates

World Obesity (2015). Global Prevalance of adult Obesity retrieved 3 October 2015 from http://www.worldobesity.com

and obese adults. See Table 23.1 for additional data on obesity in the Middle East and Gulf States.

23.2 The Qatar Experience

Hamad Medical Corporation (HMC) has been the principal public health provider in the state of Qatar for over three decades. HMC manages eight hospitals, incorporating five specialist hospitals and three Community hospitals, all accredited by Joint Commission International (JCI). HMC is leading the development of the region's first academic health system and is committed to building a legacy of health care expertise in Qatar. We collaborate with partners who are key experts in Qatar and beyond, including Weill Cornell Medical College-Qatar, Morgagni-Pierantoni Hospital, Forli, Italy, and the Institute for Healthcare Improvement and Partners HealthCare, Boston, USA.

We are also the first hospital system in the Middle East to achieve Institutional accreditation from the Accreditation Council of Graduate Medical Education International (ACGME-I), which demonstrates excellence in the way medical graduates are trained through residency, internship, and fellowship program.

Qatar Robotic Surgery Center (QRSC) works through a collaboration between Qatari and UK educational institutions whose aim is to focus on the fast-growing field of medical robotics and robotic surgery, and to promote its application in the Middle East. QRSC is committed to leading the way in the clinical application of robotic surgery in the region, and seems well on track to realize that ambition. QRSC is a focal point for international expertise in robotic surgery. The center focuses on two core activities: (1) training in robotic minimally invasive and surgical related procedures and techniques and (2) development and demonstration of innovative surgical technologies. The concept of QRSC is unique in the world, as it emphasizes on advanced simulation training and cross-fertilization between its training and technology development activities. QRSC aims to develop Qatar into a hub for robotic surgical technology, is committed to lead the way in the region in clinical application of robotic surgery and seems well on track to realize that ambition. The center is interested not only at executing research activities but also at stimulating and fostering the same with local and international partners. It targets to create a lively network of research institutions focused on surgical technologies. QRSC's in house focus areas are development of surgical skill assessment tools and techniques image guided intervention technologies and novel instrumentation.

We started our program in HMC in 2012 with collaboration of the Italian team from Morgagni-Pierantoni Hospital, Forli, Italy. To date our experience has been limited to eight patients. We believe that this number may be due to patient's refusal to undergo tracheostomy as part of the procedure. We are working to improve postoperative management in order to avoid tracheostomy in select patients in order to increase the eligibility of patients for TORS. As our program remains in its infancy we continue to focus on improving our skills through TORS courses and workshops.

We have organized TORS workshops and the surgeons who attended have had the opportunity of learning the state-of-the-art approach from the world experts, and have also had the chance to learn the fundamental principles of robotic-assisted TORS procedures including the functionality and ergonomics of da Vinci® Surgical System and its instrumentation, patient positioning, surgical team position, and surgical approaches.

23.3 Preoperative Workup

The preoperative workup is the same as previously described for OSA surgery. High risk patient should have thorough anesthesia assessment due to possible comorbidities such as uncontrolled hypertension, cardiovascular disease, arrhythmias, and pulmonary hypertension. Each patient is discussed on a case-by-case with the surgical and anesthetic team before there is a final decision to proceed with surgery.

In general, proper selection of patients for surgery is paramount to achieve successful outcomes and to minimize postoperative complications. The preoperative evaluation requires a comprehensive medical history, head and neck examination, fiber optic naso-pharyngo-laryngoscopy, and lateral cephalometry.

We usually perform a CT or MRI scan as it may help to show the degree of soft tissue collapse and to distinguish between lymphatic and muscular collapse at the base of tongue.

DISE is becoming a routine part of our preoperative evaluation of OSA as it is helpful to determine the site of obstruction. We are using either VOTE [4] or NOHL [5] classification for evaluating our OSA patients. Polysomnography remains the gold standard diagnostic test in OSA [6]. We refer all the patients to our pulmonary unit where Type 3 monitoring is usually performed. Only in selected cases is Type 1 or 2 monitoring performed.

A thorough review of this data can determine the extent of SDB severity, uncover comorbidities, and assist in risk management. Furthermore, this systemic approach will identify probable anatomic sites of obstruction. Armed with this information a safe, site-specific surgical protocol can be presented to the patient.

Airway is a very important issue to consider in OSAS surgery, because in sleep apnea surgery an already difficult airway can be further compromised by edema and bleeding. Elective tracheostomy should be planned for some medical condition as well as for some surgical indications.

Many surgeons prefer to do elective tracheostomy for severe OSAS cases s if multilevel surgery is undertaken, while mild to moderate cases who undergo limited surgery, and have reasonably good airway anatomy with limited medical comorbidities, do not need a routine tracheostomy.

The decision to perform tracheostomy at the end of the TORS case depend on several factors including neurologic status, ventilator function, upper airway patency, and presence of protective reflexes. In the initial phase of our TORS cases, we performed a tracheostomy, however we now realize that tracheostomy may be avoided in some cases [7].

23.4 Indications

The ideal patient should have significant obstruction at the tongue base, and/or prolapse of adjacent supraglottic tissue, as determined by awake endoscopy or DISE. Patient should have PSG evidence of moderate to severe OSAS.

It is well accepted that OSA surgery should not be offered to patients who are tolerant and comply with CPAP therapy, but can be offered to non-adherent patient as a primary procedure or after previous surgery failure when anatomy is appropriate.

23.5 Contraindications

Surgery should not be offered to patients who are successfully treated medically and those patients with comorbidities that result in an ASA score >3.

Local contraindications to the procedure include trismus, micrognathia, significant macroglossia with high modified Mallampati–Friedman scores and inter-incisive distance <2.5 cm.

23.6 Immediate Postoperative Management

The hospital stay has ranges between 3 and 5 days and is dependent upon a number of variables including the extent of surgery, comorbidities, pain, swallowing function, tracheostomy, and the surgeon's comfort level. Patients who have undergone multilevel surgery may need longer rehabilitation time than patients who have only had one site treated. On the first postoperative night, the patient should be monitored in a high dependency unit, not in an ordinary ward. The patient should be provided with continuous pulse oximetry, bedside suction, and should be watched closely for any bleeding or respiratory obstruction. Perioperative antibiotics and steroids should be administered.

In case of immediate postoperative bleeding the patient is returned to the operating room, the operative site inspected, and the source of bleeding cauterized and/or clipped.

References

1. Ogden CL, Carroll MD, Kit BK, Flegal KM. Prevalence of childhood and adult obesity in the United States, 2011–2012. J Am Med (JAMA). 2014;311(8):806–14.
2. Bener A, Zirie M, Janahi IM, AL-Hamaq AQ, Musallam M, Wareham NJ. Prevalance of diagnosed and undiagnosed diabetes mellitus and its risk factors in a population-based study of Qatar. Diabetes Res Clin Pract. 2009;84:99–106.
3. World Health Organization-Non communicable Diseases (NCD) country profile, Qatar 2014
4. Kezirian EJ, Hohenhorst W, de Vries N. Drug-induced sleep endoscopy: the VOTE classification. Eur Arch Otorhinolaryngol. 2011;268(8):1233–6.
5. Vicini C, De Vito A, Benazzo M, Frassineti S, Campanini A, Frasconi P, Mira E. The nose oropharynx hypopharynx and larynx (NOHL) classification: a new system of diagnostic standardized examination for OSAHS patients. Eur Arch Otorhinolaryngol. 2012;269(4):1297–300.
6. Collop NA, Anderson WM, Boehlecke B, et al. Clinical guidelines for the use of unattended portable monitors in the diagnosis of obstructive sleep apnea in adult patients. Portable Monitoring Task Force of the American Academy of Sleep Medicine. J Clin Sleep Med. 2007;3:737–47.
7. Campanini A, De Vito A, Frassineti S, Vicini C. Temporary tracheotomy in the surgical treatment of obstructive sleep apnea syndrome: personal experience. Acta Otorhinolaryngol Ital. 2003;6:474–8.

Chapter 24
The Far Eastern Asian Experience

Song Tar Toh and Vikas Agrawal

24.1 Introduction

The first case series of robotic OSAHS surgery for Asian patients was published in 2014 [1]. This modality of treatment for tongue base obstruction is established even in this group of patients with inherent disease differences compared to Caucasian patients, where TORS was initially described in 2012 [2]. Our results are similar to published results of predominantly Caucasian patients in a worldwide multicenter study [3]. The purpose of this chapter is to highlight differences seen in Asian OSA patients and how we overcome limitations with performing TORS on this group of patients and how we run our TORS program in Singapore and India.

24.2 The Asian OSA Patients

Ethnicity is known to play an important part in the pathogenesis of OSA, with underlying craniofacial skeletal differences compared to Caucasian being one of the major factors [4]. The prevalence of OSA in Asians varied according to countries (China, India, Korea, Japan, Hong Kong, Taiwan, Thailand, Malaysia, and Singapore) studied and instruments used, but it can be as low as 3.7 % to as high as 88.1 % [5].

Cephalometric analysis demonstrated that Far Eastern Asians have maxilla protrusion and mandibular retrusion (Fig. 24.1), shorter cranial base, narrower

S.T. Toh, M.B.B.S., M.M.E.D.(ORL), F.A.M.S.(ORL) (✉)
Department of Otolaryngology, Singapore General Hospital, Singapore
e-mail: songtar@gmail.com

V. Agrawal, M.S., F.C.P.S., D.O.R.L.
Department of ENT, Specialty ENT Hospital,
Satyam Tower, Thakur Complex, Kandivali East, Mumbai 400101, India

© Springer International Publishing Switzerland 2016

C. Vicini et al. (eds.), *TransOral Robotic Surgery for Obstructive Sleep Apnea*,
DOI 10.1007/978-3-319-34040-1_24

cranial base angle, larger posterior airway space, and more superiorly positioned hyoid bone compared with whites [6]. Asian OSA patients also tend to have more severe disease compared to their Caucasian counterparts after adjusting for age, gender, and body mass index (BMI) [7, 8].

Although BMI is major factor affecting Caucasian OSA patients, it has a lesser impact with majority of Asian OSA patients in the nonobese category [6–8]. Because of craniofacial restriction, mouth opening can be restricted and may impede the use of TORS, especially with the tongue in protrusion and Davis Meyer blade in situ (Fig. 24.2). This is especially so for Chinese patients. The standard 12 mm 30° up-facing camera-scope system is the workhorse of TORS. However, in Asian OSA patients, it may be necessary to use the 8.5 mm 30° camera-scope system. The view provided by the 8.5 mm 30° scope allows similar exposure of the tongue base and resection. The space gained at the teeth allow for better maneuvering of the camera system for a better view without clashing the teeth and hinging on the teeth, thus preventing teeth damage.

24.3 Pattern of Upper Airway Collapse in Asian OSA Patients

Obstructive sleep apnea is a disease characterized by repetitive multiple level airway obstruction during sleep. There is no difference in this aspect when compared to patients of other ethnicity. Before performing TORS for sleep apnea, the authors will perform drug-induced sleep endoscopy using dexmedetomidine or propofol and scored the pattern of airway obstruction using the VOTE classification [9].

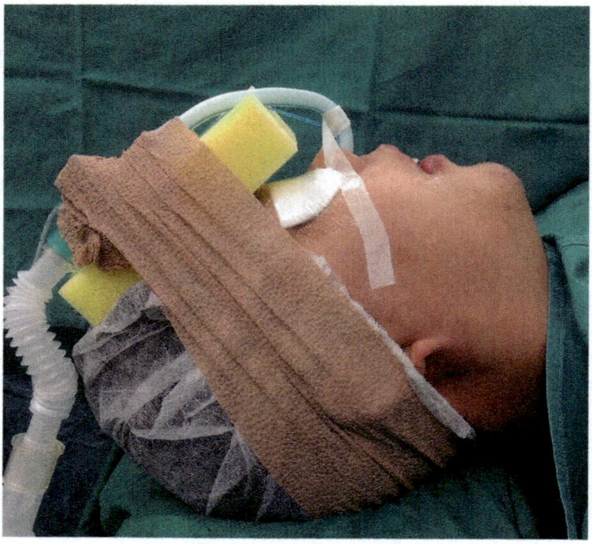

Fig. 24.1 The Asian Chinese OSA patient with mandibular retrusion

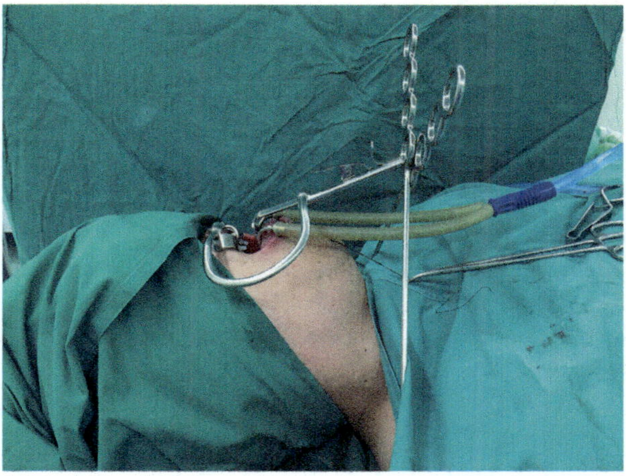

Fig. 24.2 Limited mouth opening and access for camera-scope and robotic arm

24.4 The Lingual Neurovascular Bundle in Asian Chinese OSA Patients

Because of skeletal differences between Asian and Caucasian patients, it is important before embarking on this surgical procedure to understand the anatomy of lingual neurovascular bundle in Asian patients. Studies done on Asian Chinese patients showed that the average distance between two lingual arteries at the foramen cecum of the tongue was 27.78 ± 6.57 mm, and the distance to the surface of the tongue was 29.27 ± 5.39 mm [10].

The safety area between the lingual arteries at the tongue base is stated to be about 31 mm wide with the tongue in resting position [11]. Of particular relevance is that these distances will change with changing position of the tongue during TORS with protrusion of the tongue and compression with retraction blade. A study in Asian Chinese OSA patients showed that with the tongue in the fully extended/protruded position, the depth of lingual artery to tongue dorsum and interarterial distance changed, compared to the resting position, at the foramen caecum and 1 cm before and 1 cm after the foramen caecum. The artery is brought nearer the surface at these three points (from about 28 mm to 24–25 mm) and closer together (from about 20 mm to 14 mm) at the foramen caecum [12]. Hence, the TORS robotic surgeon should be cognizant of the changes in lingual artery anatomy and safety margin during surgery for adequate resection. No such studies were available for other ethnicities.

24.5 TORS for OSA Program in Singapore and India

Singapore and India are two countries in Asia that started performing TORS for OSA. Singapore started it in 2011 and India in 2012. Currently countries like Hong Kong and Korea have also embarked on this journey. We share here our experience running our program.

24.5.1 TORS for OSA Program in Singapore

Singapore is the first country in Asia to perform transoral robotic surgery for tongue base reduction for OSA patients. The program started in Singapore General Hospital in November 2011, after we received training for the da Vinci robotic system and completed our Advanced TORS course at an Intuitive accredited robotic training center in Korea. During our Snoring and Sleep Apnea Surgery Course in early July 2013, we performed the first "Live" transoral robotic surgery for tongue base reduction for OSA, which saw Prof Claudio Vicini and Dr. Filippo Montevecchi coming as our honored guest faculty and this course was attended by 100 ENT surgeons from Asia.

It is important to create a team of dedicated surgeons, anesthesiologists, and nursing staff to ensure that the system and workflow is established and surgery is performed safely. Preoperative assessment, intraoperative care, and postoperative care in intensive care unit or high dependency unit need to be championed by respective trained staff to ensure smooth and safe surgery. Since we started, we have done close to 100 cases of TORS for tongue base reduction for OSA. In Singapore General Hospital, we followed the standard selection criteria and surgical technique, and perioperative care as outlined in the other parts of this book. We did not have to perform tracheostomy for these patients.

Majority of cases are primary palatopharyngeal reconstructive surgery combined with TORS for tongue base with the rest being TORS for tongue base reduction for patients with failed previous palatal surgeries. Our initial publication of result in 20 subjects with complete preoperative and postoperative polysomnogram showed cure rate of 35 % (AHI < 5/h) and success rate of 90 % (including cure, AHI < 20/h and 50 % reduction in AHI). For patients without postoperative polysomnographic study, subjective improvement in snoring by bed partners and Epworth sleepiness scale is observed using visual analog scale grading [1]. Both robotic set up time and robotic surgery time decrease with experience and we have reached a steady rate of 5–10 min for robotic set up time (including tongue protrusion, insertion of gag, and introduction of robotic camera and arms). The robotic surgical time is about 20–30 min. Complications include minor bleeding from tonsillar bed and base of tongue, odynophagia, poor oral feeding requiring intravenous hydration, self-limiting tongue numbness, and dysgeusia.

In our practice, we extubate the patients in the operating room and insert a nasopharyngeal airway to protect the airway. No patients required a tracheostomy or nasogastric tube feeding. The patient is then monitored in high dependency unit and given intravenous Augmentin and dexamethasone for the duration of hospitalization, which is about 2 days. We then convert to oral augmentin and dexamethasone. We also give nebulized adrenaline, normal saline, and Atrovent during the hospitalization to decreased upper airway swelling and secretion. We give paracetamol and a Cox2 inhibitor as analgesia with lozenges and gargles. We review them in the clinic in 1–2 weeks time and as needed till recovery.

24.5.2 TORS for OSA Program in India

We started the robotic surgery program for obstructive sleep apnea in September 2012 in Mumbai, and the first case was operated in December 2012. Since that time, we have come a long way in the development of the specialty and making protocols. We did the first "Live" web telecast on robotic surgery for base of tongue for ENT surgeons across the globe in July 2013, which was attended by 175 surgeons and over 2000. Our training and this course was under the guidance of Prof. Claudio Vicini from Italy.

Robotic surgery is used mainly for resection of the base of the tongue and the epiglottis. This area is critical in approximately 20 % of all OSA patients, where only palatal surgery fails to relieve obstruction. In Indian and Asian population, the role of posterior placed base of tongue is more than Caucasian population because of the facial profile. Our protocol of approach to a patient of OSA in India is similar to those outlined in this book.

We differentiate between pure lymphoid enlargement of the tongue base (lingual tonsils) and muscular enlargement of the tongue base. Lingual tonsils can be operated as daycare, as the vessels supplying lymphoid tissues are not large in caliber and can be taken care of more effectively. We also differentiate the muscular tongue base into upper tongue base collapse and lower tongue base collapse. The results of TORS in lower tongue base collapse are extremely good and we excise less amount of tissue in that area. In upper tongue base, the amount of resection is much higher to achieve the same result, and the complication rates start increasing. Maxillomandibular advancement (MMA) is considered a better suited surgery for higher tongue base collapse. Our protocol for robotic surgery for tongue base in OSA follows that of Professor Claudio Vicini that is outlined in other parts of this book.

In our practice, all patients are kept in high dependency unit postoperatively with nasotracheal intubation for 24 h to keep secure the airway in case of a respiratory compromise or unexpected bleeding. The patient is sedated with dexmeditomedine and fentanyl drip. After 24 h, the airway is examined with a flexible endoscope from the other side of the nose till the base tongue and epiglottis, before extubation is performed in semirecumbent position. The patient is kept for observation in the ward for 2–3 days with a nasogastric feeding tube, fed orally with cold water and ice creams only. Antibiotic cover is given for 3 days intravenous, then orally for 2 weeks alone with liberal use of analgesics and oral gargles. Our experience showed that outcome of the surgery is seen to be excellent in lower tongue base collapse, but not in the upper tongue base collapse.

24.6 Conclusion

Transoral robot-assisted tongue base resection for tongue base obstruction in Asian patients with obstructive sleep apnea is an established treatment modality and gives good success and cure rates, with minimal morbidity. A sleep apnea surgeon wanting to embark on this surgical modality should be cognizant of the inherent differences in disease manifestations and skeletal framework contribution compared to Caucasian patients and differences in lingual artery anatomy.

References

1. Toh ST, Han HJ, Tay HN, Kiong KL. Transoral robotic surgery for obstructive sleep apnea in Asian patients: a Singapore sleep centre experience. JAMA Otolaryngol Head Neck Surg. 2014;140(7):624–9.
2. Vicini C, Canzi P, Frassineti S, La Pietra MG, Montevecchi F. Transoral robotic tongue base resection in obstructive sleep apnoea-hypopnoea syndrome: a preliminary report. ORL J Otorhinolaryngol Relat Spec. 2010;72(1):22–7.
3. Vicini C, Montevecchi F, Campanini A, Dallan I, Hoff PT, Spector ME, Thaler E, Ahn J, Baptista P, Remacle M, Lawson G, Benazzo M, Canzi P. Clinical outcomes and complications associated with TORS for OSAHS: a benchmark for evaluating an emerging surgical technology in a targeted application for benign disease. ORL J Otorhinolaryngol Relat Spec. 2014;76(2):63–9.
4. Lee W, Nagubadi S, Kryger MH, Mokhlesi B. Epidemiology of obstructive sleep apnea: a population-based perspective. Expert Rev Respir Med. 2008;2(3):349–64.
5. Mirrakhimov AE, Sooronbaev T, Mirrakhimov EM. Prevalence of obstructive sleep apnea in Asian adults: a systematic review of the literature. BMC Pulm Med. 2013;13:10.
6. Li KK, Powell NB, Kushida C, Riley RW, Adornato B, Guilleminault C. A comparison of Asian and white patients with obstructive sleep apnea syndrome. Laryngoscope. 1999;109(12):1937–40.
7. Ong KC, Clerk AA. Comparison of the severity of sleep-disordered breathing in Asian and Caucasian patients seen at a sleep disorders center. Respir Med. 1998;92:843–8.
8. Li KK, Kushida C, Adornato B, et al. Obstructive sleep apnea syndrome in the Asian population. Sleep. 1999;22:S104.
9. Kezirian EJ, Hohenhorst W, de Vries N. Drug-induced sleep endoscopy: the VOTE classification. Eur Arch Otorhinolaryngol. 2011;268(8):1233–6.
10. Li SH, Shi HJ. Lingual artery CTA-guided midline partial glossectomy for treatment of obstructive sleep apnea hypopnea syndrome. Acta Otolaryngol. 2013;133(7):749–54.
11. Hou T, Shao J, Fang S. The definition of the V zone for the safety space of functional surgery of the tongue. Laryngoscope. 2012;122(1):66–70.
12. Wu DH, Qin J, Guo XH, Li SH. Analysis of the difference in the course of the lingual arteries caused by tongue position change. Laryngoscope. 2015;125:762–6.

Chapter 25
The Australian Experience

Suren Krishnan and Julia A. Crawford

25.1 Introduction

There are few studies looking at the prevalence of sleep disorders in Australia, but an evaluation of the sleep habits of Australians found that 20–35 % of the population suffered from disrupted sleep, inadequate sleep duration, daytime fatigue, excessive sleepiness and irritability with the most common diagnosed sleep disorder being OSAS [1].

In 2010 approximately 4.7 % of the Australian population overall were affected by OSA; 6.4 % of males and 3.6 % of females. The importance of sleep health is gaining increased recognition as both the personal and societal costs are better understood. Sleep disorders cost the hospital system around $96.2 million but imposes a burden that extends far beyond the diagnosis and treatment of the disorders themselves [2].

The associated cost encompasses medical conditions that occur as a consequence of suffering OSA such as the increased risk of hypertension, stroke, myocardial infarction and depression. However there are also substantial indirect financial and non-financial costs involved. Other financial costs include the common consequences of insufficient sleep such as the costs of work-related injuries, motor vehicle accidents and productivity losses. Non-financial costs are related to the loss of quality of life and premature death that is associated with long-term severe sleep disorders [3].

S. Krishnan, M.B.B.S., F.R.A.C.S. (✉)
Department of Otolaryngology, Head and Neck Surgery, Royal Adelaide Hospital,
Adelaide, SA, Australia
e-mail: krishnan.suren@gmail.com

J.A. Crawford, B.Sc., M.B.B.S., F.R.A.C.S.
Department of Otolaryngology, Head and Neck Surgery, St. Vincent's Hospital,
Darlinghurst, NSW, Australia

© Springer International Publishing Switzerland 2016

C. Vicini et al. (eds.), *TransOral Robotic Surgery for Obstructive Sleep Apnea*,
DOI 10.1007/978-3-319-34040-1_25

In Australia, the gold standard for treatment of OSA remains the use of continuous positive airway pressure (CPAP), but there has been increasing research into surgical alternatives with good results [4].

25.2 History of TORS in Australia

The application of TORS for the treatment of OSA is still in its infancy in Australia.

The first surgical robot was installed at Epworth Private Hospital in Melbourne in 2003 and the second was installed in Adelaide at the Royal Adelaide Hospital in 2003. By 2007 there were five da Vinci® robots (Intuitive Surgical, Sunnyvale, CA) across four states. This number dramatically rose to more than 25 within 10 years.

The Royal Adelaide Hospital was the first hospital to perform TORS in Australia in July 2008. This hospital is a public hospital and has now performed some 250 TORS procedures. The majority of procedures are for oropharyngeal cancer and include lateral oropharyngectomy and tongue base resections. The case load includes partial and total laryngectomy and resection of parapharyngeal space tumours as well as experience with TORS assisted neck dissection.

There are now robotically trained surgeons in most Australian states and the expertise continues to rise as surgeons who are fellowship trained in robotic surgery return to practice in Australia.

25.3 The Royal Adelaide Experience

The Royal Adelaide Hospital has performed 20 procedures for OSA using the da Vinci® surgical robot. These procedures are limited in number because the service is provided in a public hospital system. There is limited access to this resource and its use is prioritized for use in patients with cancer.

The use of TORS has been justified in patients with OSA because these patients were considered to have difficult transoral access. This is comparable to the reported 18.6 % of 182 consecutive OSAS cases with difficult access and difficult intubation at Stanford [5].

We have used the robot for a variety of surgical procedures described for OSA [6]. Our experience suggests that the da Vinci® robot is a useful device in accessing and performing surgery in patients with OSA. The surgical procedures performed include a palatal using a variety of techniques, expansion pharyngoplasty and palatal advancement as well as the recently described double barbed uvulopalatopharyngoplasty. We have also used TORS for tongue volume reduction surgery including tongue base lingual tonsillectomy, tongue base excision and submucosal, minimally invasive lingual excision (SMILE) [6].

Although our experience is not randomised and controlled, our results demonstrate a benefit in the use of TORS for OSA. All our patients improved with 50 % reduction in RDI after surgery and all improved symptomatically. We had one post-operative bleed on day 4 return to theatre and one planned pre-operative tracheostomy.

The experience at the Royal Adelaide Hospital has been with the use of three da Vinci surgical robot systems; the original standard® system, the da Vinci S® and the new Xi® system. Our experience has included the use of 5 and 8 mm instruments, but our preference has been to use the 8 mm instruments. The new Xi® system provides excellent optical and instrument access to perform oropharyngeal surgery for OSA and in our opinion is a definitive technological advance.

There is no recorded use of TORS for OSA in other centres in Australia at the time of this report.

References

1. Mansfield DR, McEvoy RD. Sleep disorders: a practical guide for Australian health care practitioners. MJA Suppl. 2013;199(8):S1–40.
2. Deloitte Access Economics. Re-awakening Australia: the economic cost of sleep disorders in Australia, 2010. Canberra, Australia: Deloitte Access Economics; 2011. http://www.sleephealthfoundation.org.au/pdfs/news/Reawakenings%20Australia.pdf. Accessed Oct 2015.
3. Hillman DR, Murphy AS, Antic R, Pezzulo L. The economic costs of sleep disorders. Sleep. 2006;29:299–305.
4. Mackay SG, Carney A, Woods C, Antic N, McEvoy R, Chia M, Sands T, Jones A, Hobson J, Robinson S. Modified uvulopalatopharyngoplasty and coblation channeling of the tongue for obstructive sleep apnea: a multi-centre Australian trial. J Clin Sleep Med. 2013;9(2):117–24.
5. Riley R, Powell N, Guilleminault C. Obstructive sleep apnea syndrome: a review of 306 consecutively treated surgical patients. Otolaryngol Head Neck Surg. 1993;108:117–25.
6. Robinson S, Krishnan S, Hodge J, Foreman A. Robot-assisted, volumetric tongue base reduction and pharyngeal surgery for obstructive sleep apnea. Oper Tech Otolaryngol. 2012;23(1):48–55.

Part V
Research and Future Perspectives

Chapter 26
Research and Future Perspectives

Claudio Vicini, Filippo Montevecchi, Paul T. Hoff, Asit Arora, and E. Vetri

26.1 Introduction

Following the introduction of TORS for base of tongue neoplasms [1], sleep surgeons quickly recognized the applicability of lingual tonsillectomy and base of tongue resection for the treatment of OSA [2]. Early retrospective clinical studies demonstrated safety and efficacy which culminated in the Food and Drug Administration (FDA) approval of TORS for resection of benign tissue from the base of tongue [3]; however, an endorsement of TORS for the specific clinical indication of OSA was not given.

The immediate goal of the sleep surgery community is to obtain FDA approval through a prospective clinical trial demonstrating safety and efficacy of TORS-assisted multilevel surgery for moderate-to-severe OSA.

Patient selection remains an inexact science. Investigators have demonstrated predictors of success including BMI, Friedman stage, and lingual tonsil volume (Spector et al., unpublished, D'Agostino, unpublished) [4]. Hopefully in the near

C. Vicini, M.D. • F. Montevecchi, M.D.
Head and Neck Department - ENT & Oral Surgery Unit - G.B. Morgagni - L. Pierantoni Hospital, Forlì – Infermi Hospital, Faenza - ASL of Romagna, Italy
e-mail: claudio@claudiovicini.com; filo651@hotmail.com; filippomontevecchi72@gmail.com

P.T. Hoff, M.S., M.D.
Department of Otolaryngology–Head and Neck Surgery, University of Michigan Health System, Ann Arbor, MI, USA

A. Arora, Ph.D., D.I.C., F.R.C.S.
Department of Otorhinolaryngology and Head & Neck Surgery, St. Mary's Hospital, Imperial College Healthcare NHS Trust, London, UK

E. Vetri, M.D.
Medical Direction, G.B. Morgagni—L. Pierantoni Hospital,
Via Carlo Forlanini, 34, 47121 Forlì, Italy
e-mail: elena.vetri@auslromagna.it

© Springer International Publishing Switzerland 2016

C. Vicini et al. (eds.), *TransOral Robotic Surgery for Obstructive Sleep Apnea*,
DOI 10.1007/978-3-319-34040-1_26

future a more comprehensive evaluation of patients by means of new tools of anatomic and functional phenotype characterization will help for a better selection of the proper surgical candidates. The role of sleep endoscopy to further enhance our ability to predict surgical success or failure and type of surgery to be performed is an area of active investigation. New interesting tools are under intensive investigation, including a new stratification of OSA patients in terms of phenotypic traits as obtained by a complex PSG/CPAP experimental setting devised by Edwards and Wellman [5] in Boston. When the system becomes available for commercial use it could be an additional tool for improving patient selection for surgery including TORS.

We are now in a golden era for OSA-related treatment options. Patients may now choose between CPAP, positional therapy, oral appliance therapy, bariatric surgery, hypoglossal nerve stimulation, and a multitude of surgical treatments including TORS for base of tongue obstruction. The day is approaching when surgical treatment may be considered first-line therapy in highly selected adult patient with OSA just as it has been in pediatric OSA patients for decades [6].

TORS for OSA is in its infancy. Future treatment options for OSA are in a state of rapid evolution. The role of CPAP remains the foundation; however many innovations, both nonsurgical and surgical, are expanding options for patients. TORS offers a new surgical modality to affect changes in tongue base obstruction. TORS for OSA is the final step in a comprehensive assessment of patient anatomy, comorbidities, and expectations. The intent of this chapter is to outline specific areas where future work will lead to the final evolution of multilevel treatment for OSA including:

1. Patient selection
2. Drug-induced sedation endoscopy (DISE)
3. Advanced technology
4. Refinement of surgical technique
5. Salvage surgery
6. Outcome research
7. Pathophysiology
8. Economics

26.2 Patient Selection

The ultimate goal of surgery is to provide patients with a predictable outcome with an acceptable risk of unfavorable outcomes. The surgeon's dream is to have a perfect diagnostic tool for selecting the patient who will be fixed by the procedure and exclude those patients who will fail or will develop serious complications. There are currently no universally accepted selection criteria for TORS multilevel surgery. There have been a number of papers showing that success is dependent upon BMI, Friedman stage, and lingual tonsil volume; however, every surgeon has anecdotal reports of success in patients outside of these parameters. The awake and obstructed airway is complex and highly individualized. As a result many surgeons do not have a strict cutoff for BMI and lingual tonsil volume resection varies from patient to patient; many surgeons do not measure resected volume.

Although we are moving toward a better understanding of the anatomic features that predict surgical outcomes, we are just beginning to understand and manipulate the dynamic neurophysiology involved in airway maintenance during wakefulness and sleep. As for in many other surgical areas a multicenter study or hopefully an international common database would be of great interest in order to define a sound predictive success index.

Only in the last 2 years there have been attempts to use DISE to predict success or failure. Further work needs to be done to integrate anthropometric findings, cephalometrics, Friedman staging, preoperative imaging (MRI), genioglossal muscle EMG, and DISE to arrive upon a comprehensive staging system that will give sleep surgeons the confidence to offer surgery with a predictable outcome. This staging system would not be unlike the TNM staging system for head and neck cancer patients.

26.3 Drug-Induced Sedated Endoscopy

Since Fujuta [7] began performing UPPP in the 1980s, surgeons have struggled to predict successful outcomes in their patients. The advent of DISE in 1991 heralded an innovative method to study the obstructed airway during sleep. Since Croft and Pringle's original description of DISE five different classification systems have been introduced. In 2014 the European Position Paper on DISE [8] reached significant consensus with the exception of a universal classification system and a method for standardized scoring of data.

DISE has been found to be more effective than in office Mueller maneuver at detecting collapse with only 30 % agreement in findings. In addition DISE is able to identify areas of collapse in the hypopharynx and epiglottis not seen during awake examination.

Only in the last 2 years there have been attempts to use DISE to predict success or failure. For example, the presence of concentric collapse in the velum was a negative predictor of success in the start trial for hypoglossal nerve stimulation; these patients were eliminated from consideration of treatment.

Using DISE, Kezirian [9] found that the majority of non-responders to pharyngeal surgery for OSA showed residual palatal obstruction and almost all had hypopharyngeal obstruction. Thaler et al. [10] are combining DISE findings with objective dynamic MRI imaging, and anthropometric data to best predict treatment success and treatment failure. The International Sleep Surgery Society under the leadership of Kezirian is currently gathering DISE data from major centers from around the world in an effort to create a database for future investigation of DISE and its role in the evaluation of patients with OSA.

In 2014 a new and exciting chapter of the OSA evaluation was introduced by a group in Boston [5]. The concept of functional phenotypization by means of a sophisticated modified CPAP may allow investigators to obtain an increasing amount of information about the loop gain, arousal threshold, critical pressure, etc. From the surgical point of view, phenotypization basically means the possibility to correlate a functional profile with a probability of surgical success. Currently, this approach is still too complicated for routine clinical use; however more simplified and practical solutions are under evaluation.

DISE also plays a key role in the evaluation of patients undergoing evaluation for salvage surgery.

26.4 Advanced Technology

A new generation of robotic tools may be dedicated for OSA surgery and perhaps revolutionary robotic systems may be on the horizon. New instrumentation including retractors and blades will improve exposure, and alternative cutting devices may improve postoperative morbidity. A navigation system may allow surgeons to plan and carry out surgery with more precision. Tissue-specific dyes will be available for easier intraoperative identification of nerves and vessels.

The current da Vinci Si® platform has served the first generation of TORS sleep surgeons well. Many surgeons continue to use an earlier generation S model with great success. Rarely does the surgeon encounter a patient with trismus or micrognathia that precludes TORS with either the S or Si model. One could argue that patients who have such unfavorable anatomy would be poor candidates for surgical treatment of OSA. That being said, there are exciting new technologies on the horizon including non-robotic video-assisted procedures that may have widespread appeal due to affordability and possibly decreased morbidity.

Can we do a better job with postoperative pain control and wound healing with an alternative energy source? The standard cutting tool provided with the da Vinci® system is a spatula monopolar cautery. Even at a low-energy setting, monopolar cautery causes collateral thermal injury. Alternative energy sources that are familiar to head and neck surgeons include Harmonic Scalpel® and cold ablation (Coblation®). Technology that has been used with the robot in the past includes the thulium laser and the CO_2 laser but have not found widespread acceptance due to the inability to dual purpose the cutting instrument as a dissector.

The da Vinci Single Port® is a natural evolution in robotic surgery to access areas including the skull base (transnasal), parapharyngeal space, or glottic larynx. Although this technology is very interesting, it may not offer the surgeon much of an advantage when working on the tongue base for OSA. Patients with a small oral aperture or macroglossia are unlikely to have good clinical outcomes with surgery, whether it is performed with the Single Port, Si, or even the Chabolle procedure.

Competitors in TORS platforms have recently come to the market; the Medrobotics Flex System® has recently demonstrated safety and efficacy in a small study from

Belgium where base of tongue and lingual tonsillectomy were performed for OSA [11]. Fortunately our surgical armamentarium continues to expand in other areas including hypoglossal nerve stimulation so that those patients who seek alternatives to CPAP do have options. Surgeons with a variety of tools may be able to offer combined techniques incorporating soft-tissue resection or skeletal framework surgery, neuromodulation, or other modalities (positional therapy, oral appliance therapy) to achieve the ultimate goal of patient satisfaction and successful treatment of OSA.

26.5 Refinement of Surgical Technique

It's advisable to develop more customized techniques for the individual patients according to the recognized obstruction sites and patterns. Combining our knowledge of anatomy with dynamic collapse as seen with DISE and imaging (MRI, cephalometrics) has already led to targeted surgical procedures. Further refinement is needed as our overall success rate remains under 80 %. Development of a preoperative algorithm that will predict success or failure is perhaps the next major hurdle to be crossed. When surgical outcomes become predictable it would be reasonable to follow Rotenberg's suggestion that surgery can supplant CPAP as first-line treatment in highly selected patients [12].

So far TORS for OSA was applied mainly to the tongue base area. But pharyngeal tongue and oral tongue are a single anatomical organ, and in some cases oral tongue may represent the main obstructing pathology or may contribute in a significant way to the overall obstruction. An increased attention to this overlooked issue prompted some authors to work in the area of developing a more flexible strategy including midline oral tongue resection with the use of customized blades.

Areas of ongoing concern include postoperative morbidity. Work is being done to address postoperative pain and dysphagia through two different approaches: alternative energy sources and enhanced postoperative pharmacologic pain management.

Collateral damage due to thermal injury has long been an issue with monopolar cautery. The current surgical robotic platform is equipped with monopolar cautery; it is at the surgeon's discretion as to the energy settings used during dissection which can vary from cut, blended, and cautery modes at settings from 10 to 30 J. The amount of collateral damage will vary with each technique. Some authors report anecdotal improved pain scores with the use of CO_2 laser and thulium laser. Goh and co-workers have recently reported on their experience with Coblation® technology and video-assisted transoral endoscopic tongue base surgery. Other techniques that may offer improved pain outcomes include harmonic scalpel and bipolar cautery coupled with microdebrider. Cryosurgery could also find application in the treatment of lingual tonsil hypertrophy.

The ease of dissection with monopolar cautery has led many authors away from Coblation® and laser technology. Controlling postoperative pain has become a focus of attention; however little has been published in this area. Reports on the use of perioperative gabapentin have been promising; however our own experience with this medication in conjunction with regular-visiting home nursing resulted in a doubling of our readmission rate. We speculate that the increased rate of admission was due to the new factor of home nurses with a low threshold for advising admission to the emergency department for rehydration; further study of gabapentin is warranted. The use of cyclooxygenase-2 (COX-2) inhibitors has become more prevalent and does not appear to cause an increased risk of postoperative bleeding. Finally, there is considerable interest in new long-acting local analgesics; liposomal bupivacaine has been FDA approved for postoperative pain control following hernia repair but has not been approved for intraoral injection. This medication has a local active time of 3 days which would be a considerable benefit in the recovery following TORS.

Specific surgical refinements include targeted surgical techniques and combined modality strategies. Thaler et al. [13] have recently shown that the use of a limited excision of lateral pharyngeal wall tissue during TORS multilevel surgery including base of tongue reduction had a marked increase in success rate compared to similar historical controls (67 % vs. 30 %).

The patient's ambition to be free of CPAP must be met with realistic surgical goals. In some cases patients can be successfully managed with single-modality treatment (e.g., multilevel surgery). In other cases combined modality treatment may be a reasonable alternative; this may include surgery followed by oral appliance therapy. Recent advances with hypoglossal nerve stimulation may offer a new mode of combined therapy—lymphoid tissue reduction followed by hypoglossal nerve stimulation.

26.6 Outcome Research

TORS for OSA remains in its infancy. There remains a paucity of published data and long-term outcomes are unknown. Beginning with the first publication [2], there have been approximately 1200 patients discussed in the literature and 28 papers published in the English literature between 2010 and 2015 (Fig. 26.1).

Centers embarking on a TORS for OSA program should strongly consider collecting data in an effort to better understand both clinical sleep outcomes and short- and long-term morbidity as well as economic data. The authors recommend that surgeons performing TORS for OSA consider collecting the following data:

1. Quality of life data:
   a. Functional outcome of sleepiness questionnaire—short form (FOSQ 10) [14]
   b. Epworth Sleepiness scale (ESS) [15]
2. Swallowing function
   a. MD Anderson Dysphagia Index (MDADI) [16]

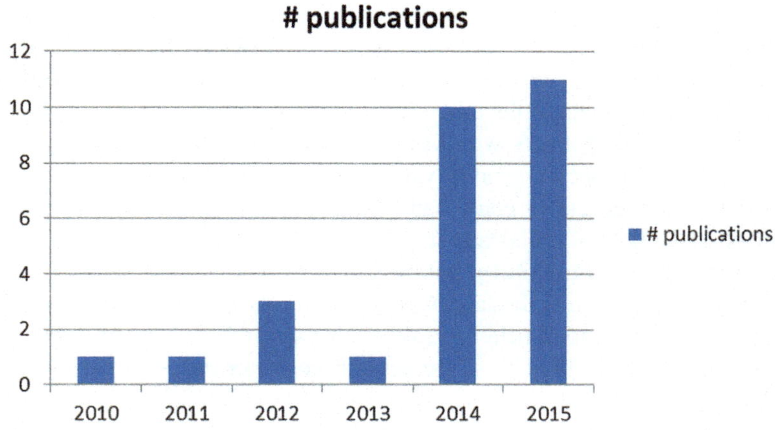

Fig. 26.1 Papers published on TORS for OSAS

3. Beyond AHI
   a. Percent time O_2 under 90 %
   b. Oxygen desaturation index (ODI)
   c. Pre- and post-treatment blood pressure
4. Economic data
   a. Robot time
   b. Length of stay
   c. Complications

Readmission rate

Serious adverse events

26.7 Salvage Surgery

Despite refinements in surgical technique, as more patients undergo surgical treatment for OSA, there will be a subset of patients who will fail and salvage procedures will become more important. Palate failures and tongue base failures will require a comprehensive set of surgical options to allow the surgeon to improve outcomes.

DISE and other anthropometric measures play an important role in the evaluation of failed surgery. Kezirian [9] identified sites of failure at the level of the velum and tongue base following UPPP.

The surgeon has to be very careful about offering additional surgery when previous attempts have failed. There are two general categories of surgical failure:

1. Failure after single-level surgery
2. Failure after multilevel surgery

Patients who fail after single-level surgery (Fujita stage 1) are often good candidates for salvage as long as preoperative predictors of success are carefully assessed and preoperative DISE is performed. Many of these patients may have undergone UPPP without assessment of the tongue base and epiglottis.

In our experience patients who have failed previous multilevel surgery with TORS who then undergo surgical salvage have a success rate under 50 % ($n=10$). Of those who are successful many had residual lingual tonsil tissue that was not recognized at the time of initial surgery.

A different subset of multilevel failures are those who underwent prior radiofrequency ablation of the tongue base, Coblation®, or suspension procedures. These patients will likely respond better to salvage because the volume of lingual tonsil tissue remaining will be high in most cases. Anecdotal evidence would suggest that the risk of functional complications (dysphagia and dysgeusia) increases with each additional procedure; this is an area worthy of further investigation. It is highly recommended that preoperative DISE be performed in all patients being considered for primary or salvage TORS.

26.8 Pathophysiology

What is the pathophysiology of lingual tonsil hypertrophy? Investigators are actively working on a better understanding of the cause of lingual tonsil hypertrophy, neuroregulation of the pharyngeal dilators, and fat accumulation in the oropharynx.

Does compensatory lingual tonsil hypertrophy occur secondary to palatine and adenoid tonsillectomy? Guttman et al. [17] found a dramatic increase in lingual tonsil hypertrophy (73 %) patients who underwent previous tonsillectomy compared to age-matched controls who did not undergo previous tonsillectomy (34 %). Although this was a small series (48 patients in each group) the findings are compelling.

HPV? This is an area of active interest. HPV lives deep in the crypts of the lingual tonsils. The sequence of events linked to the oncologic change manifesting as basaloid squamous cell carcinoma may begin with lymphoid hyperplasia. If HPV expression is causing lingual tonsil hypertrophy, is it possible that the HPV vaccination with the tetravalent vaccine will lead to the elimination of OSA in a subset of patients with massive lingua tonsil hypertrophy?

Ongoing research into the role of laryngopharyngeal reflux and lingual tonsil hypertrophy continues to yield compelling results suggesting that GERD may be a contributing factor [18–20]. Others are investigating the role of hormonal influence on the lymphoid tissue in Waldeyer's ring [21]. One cannot help but wonder if a component of OSA—lymphoid hyperplasia—may be amenable to pharmacologic or immune modulation in the form of vaccination. The obesity epidemic is a health care crisis and contributes enormously to the increased prevalence of OSA; however obesity is not related to lymphoid hypertrophy. Obesity has been found to be a negative predictor of success for multilevel surgery with TORS [4].

26.9 Economics

In an era of run-away health care costs do we have a less expensive alternative to TORS? The cost of robotic surgery is not borne by otolaryngologists alone. TORS is typically a small portion of a larger robotic program at most institutions. Colleagues in urology, gynecology, colorectal surgery, thoracic surgery, and cardiac surgery are heavy users of minimally invasive robotic surgery techniques. At many institutions the percentage of robot time allocated to otolaryngology for TORS procedures (primarily sleep related) is much less than other surgical specialities.

The cost of TORS however cannot be underestimated particularly at institutions contemplating purchase of a robot for otolaryngology alone. The economics of robotic surgery dictate that in order to be financially feasible 250 cases need to be performed annually. The cost of disposable instruments for TORS is minimal requiring only a monopolar cautery and Maryland dissector. The maintenance costs are a fixed expense regardless the number of cases. Low-volume utilizers will have higher cost for each case.

TORS gives us excellent exposure and control at a high price. Similarly, we are able to obtain adequate exposure with video-assisted tongue base surgery. Is exposure good enough for OSA? With further study, it may be possible that Coblation® or monopolar cautery using 30° scope and a Davis Meyer® mouth gag for exposure may show an equivalence or at least an acceptable success rate. Patients around the world would benefit from this prudent evolution of multilevel surgery. As our understanding of patient selection for OSA surgery improves, more patients will seek out surgical treatment for OSA. The demand for surgery will not just be in first-world countries but also in less developed areas of the world. It is incumbent upon the surgical sleep community to design treatment that is accessible to all.

References

1. O'Malley Jr BW, Weinstein GS, Snyder W, Hockstein NG. Transoral robotic surgery (TORS) for base of tongue neoplasms. Laryngoscope. 2006;116(8):1465–72.
2. Vicini C, Dallan I, Canzi P, Frassineti S, La Pietra MG, Montevecchi F. Transoral robotic tongue base resection in obstructive sleep apnoea-hypopnoea syndrome: a preliminary report. ORL J Otorhinolaryngol Relat Spec. 2010;72(1):22–7.
3. Hoff PT, D'Agostino MA, Thaler ER. Transoral robotic surgery in benign diseases including obstructive sleep apnea: safety and feasibility. Laryngoscope. 2015;125(5):1249–53.
4. Hoff PT, Glazer TA, Spector ME. Body mass index predicts success in patients undergoing transoral robotic surgery for obstructive sleep apnea. ORL J Otorhinolaryngol Relat Spec. 2014;76(5):266–72.
5. Edwards BA, Wellman A, Sands SA, Owens RL, Eckert DJ, White DP, Malhotra A. Obstructive sleep apnea in older adults is a distinctly different physiological phenotype. Sleep. 2014;37(7):1227–36. doi:10.5665/sleep.3844.
6. Pang KP, Rotenberg BW. Redefining successful therapy in obstructive sleep apnea: a call to arms. Laryngoscope. 2014;124(5):1051–2.
7. Fujita S. UPPP for sleep apnea and snoring. Ear Nose Throat J. 1984;63(5):227–35.

8. De Vito A, Carrasco Llatas M, Agnoletti V, et al. European position paper on drug-induced sedation endoscopy (DISE). Sleep Breath. 2014;18(3):453–65.
9. Kezirian EJ. Nonresponders to pharyngeal surgery for obstructive sleep apnea: insights from drug-induced sleep endoscopy. Laryngoscope. 2011;121(6):1320–6.
10. Chiffer RC, Schwab RJ, Keenan BT, Borek RC, Thaler ER. Volumetric MRI analysis pre- and post-transoral robotic surgery for obstructive sleep apnea. Laryngoscope. 2015;125(8):1988–95.
11. Remacle M, M N Prasad V, Lawson G, Plisson L, Bachy V, Van der Vorst S. Transoral robotic surgery (TORS) with the Medrobotics Flex™ System: first surgical application on humans. Eur Arch Otorhinolaryngol. 2015;272(6):1451–5.
12. Rotenberg BW, Theriault J, Gottesman S. Redefining the timing of surgery for obstructive sleep apnea in anatomically favorable patients. Laryngoscope. 2014;124 Suppl 4:S1–9.
13. Thaler ER, Rassekh CH, Lee JM, Weinstein GS, O'Malley Jr BW. Outcomes for multilevel surgery for sleep apnea: obstructive sleep apnea, transoral robotic surgery, and uvulopalatopharyngoplasty. Laryngoscope. 2015 Jul 7. doi:10.1002/lary.25353 [Epub ahead of print].
14. Weaver TE, Laizner AM, Evans LK, Maislin G, Chugh DK, Lyon K, Smith PL, Schwartz AR, Redline S, Pack AI, Dinges DF. An instrument to measure functional status outcomes for disorders of excessive sleepiness. Sleep. 1997;20(10):835–43.
15. Johns MW. A new method for measuring daytime sleepiness: the Epworth sleepiness scale. Sleep. 1991;14(6):540–5.
16. Gillespie MB, Brodsky MB, Day TA, Lee FS, Martin-Harris B. Swallowing-related quality of life after head and neck cancer treatment. Laryngoscope. 2004;114(8):1362–7.
17. Guttman D, Shvero J. Lingual tonsil hypertrophy in patients with a history of palatine tonsillectomy. Med Con. 2014;4(36):43–5.
18. Sung MW, Lee WH, Wee JH, Lee CH, Kim E, Kim JW. Factors associated with hypertrophy of the lingual tonsils in adults with sleep-disordered breathing. JAMA Otolaryngol Head Neck Surg. 2013;139(6):598–603.
19. Hwang MS, Salapatas AM, Yalamanchali S, Joseph NJ, Friedman M. Factors associated with hypertrophy of the lingual tonsils. Otolaryngol Head Neck Surg. 2015;152(5):851–5.
20. DelGaudio JM, Naseri I, Wise JC. Proximal pharyngeal reflux correlates with increasing severity of lingual tonsil hypertrophy. Otolaryngol Head Neck Surg. 2008;138(4):473–8.
21. Liu X, Liu J, Yang X, Zhang L, Wang G. Plasma estrogen level and estrogen receptors expression in palatine tonsils in male patients with obstructive sleep apnea hypopnea syndrome. Zhonghua Er Bi Yan Hou Tou Jing Wai Ke Za Zhi. 2014;49(11):920–4 [Article in Chinese].

Index

A
AASM. *See* American Association of Sleep Medicine (AASM)
AFOI. *See* Awake fiber-optic intubation (AFOI)
AHI. *See* Apnea hypopnea index (AHI)
Airway management, 140
  AFOI, 112
  direct laryngoscopy *vs.* video laryngoscopy, 111–112
  GlideScope® video laryngoscope, 111, 112
  preoxygenation, 110
  tracheal intubation (DI), 111
American Association of Sleep Medicine (AASM), 22, 23
American Society of Anesthesiology (ASA), 145
Anterior midline glossectomy, 134
Apnea, 1
Apnea Hypopnea Index (AHI), 1, 21, 146, 147
Aquaplast®, 154
Ascending palatine artery (ApaA), 93, 94
Ascending pharyngeal artery (APA), 93, 94
Asian Chinese OSA patient, 204
Asian OSA Patients, 203–204
Australian experience
  financial costs, 209
  sleep disorders, 209
  TORS, Australia, 210
Awake fiber-optic intubation (AFOI), 112

B
Barbed reposition pharyngoplasty (BRP), 74
Basaloid squamous cell carcinoma, 222
Base of tongue (BOT)
  blood supply, 100–101
  DISE, 64, 65
  HLNVB, 67
  hypoglossal nerve, 102
  LN, 102
  oropharyngeal stenosis, 67
  OSAHS, 63
  sleep endoscopy, 63
  surgical technique, 65–66
BBOTR. *See* Benign base of tongue resection (BBOTR)
Benign base of tongue resection (BBOTR), 146
BIS. *See* Bispectral Index monitoring® (BIS)
BIS®, 42
Bispectral Index monitoring® (BIS), 114
Body mass index (BMI)
  OSAHS, 56, 57
BOT. *See* Base of tongue (BOT)
Brazilian experience, 183–185

C
Cephalometry
  bony and soft tissue structures, 34
  H-MP, 34
  MMA, 34
  skeletal craniofacial morphology, 34
Chabolle's operation, 78–79
  Inspire® and Apnex®, 81
  transcervical suprahyoid approach, 78
Coblation®, 2
Coblation® technology, 219

© Springer International Publishing Switzerland 2016

C. Vicini et al. (eds.), *TransOral Robotic Surgery for Obstructive Sleep Apnea*,
DOI 10.1007/978-3-319-34040-1

Complication management
bleeding, 153
digastric and mylohyoid muscles, 153
hemostasis, 153
hypoglossal nerve, 153
immediate postoperative complications, 154–155
intra-oral trauma, 154
lingual artery arises, 153
monopolar cautery, 155
multicentric study, 155
OSAHS surgery, 151
suction-monopolar diathermy device, 155
trans-oral anatomy, 152
Computed tomography (CT)
3D MDCT analysis, 35
hypopharyngeal endoscopic evaluation, 36
CPAP, 115, 170
Crowe-Davis® mouth gag, 87
CT. *See* Computed Tomography (CT)

D
da Vinci robotic surgery, 183
da Vinci® Surgical System, 84, 121, 218
Davis Meyer® mouth gag, 122
Davis-Meyer® blades (Karl Storz), 87, 88
Dessi® (Microfrance), 123
Diet, 141
Dingman®, 87
Drug induced sleep endoscopy (DISE)
BOT level, 64
Drug-induced sedation endoscopy (DISE)
anteroposterior pattern, 47, 49
coexisting hypopharyngeal collapse, 42
hypopharyngeal and laryngeal obstruction, 47, 48
hypopharyngeal obstruction, 217
NOHL score, 47, 48
pediatric bronchoscope, 44
phenotypization, 218
Propofol®, 43
PSG, 41
SDB, 44
supraglottic collapse, 46
Dysgeusia, 163
Dysphagia
aspiration, 159
epiglottoplasty, 160
midline anterior glossectomy/palatal surgeries, 161
nasogastric feeding tube, 163
odynophagia, 163
sleep apnea, 160
swallowing, 161
tongue base, 160
tracheostomy, 163
transoral robotic surgery, 164
upper aerodigestive tracts, 159

E
ECA. *See* External carotid artery (ECA)
Efficacy
AHI, 147
definition, 146, 147
systolic hypertension, 148
Endo Wrist®, 84, 122
Endoscopy, 13, 14
Epiglottis, 189, 191
Epiglottoplasty, 130–132, 134
ESP. *See* Expansion sphincter pharyngoplasty (ESP)
Expansion sphincter pharyngoplasty (ESP), 73
External carotid artery (ECA)
ascending pharyngeal artery, 98
facial artery, 97

F
Failures management
ICSD-3, 167
LAUP, 170, 171
physical examination, 168
POSA, 168, 169
sleep endoscopy, 169–170
Feyh-Kastenbauer-Weinstein-O'Malley (FK-WO®) retractor (Olympus), 66, 87
Fiber-optic nasoendoscopy, 161
FOSQ. *See* Functional Outcome of Sleepiness Questionnaire (FOSQ)
Friedman staging system, 55–56
Functional Outcome of Sleepiness Questionnaire (FOSQ), 148

G
Gastrostomy tube, 141
Genioglossus advancement (GGA), 2, 79–80
GlideScope® video laryngoscope, 111, 112
Goettingen® retractor, 87, 88
Goettingen® table, 85, 86

H
Hamad Medical Corporation (HMC), 198
Hemostasis, 153

HLNVB. *See* Hypoglossal/lingual artery neurovascular bundle (HLNVB)
HMC. *See* Hamad Medical Corporation (HMC)
H-MP. *See* Hyoid bone and mandibular plane (H-MP)
Hyoglossus muscle (HG, 9
Hyoid bone and mandibular plane (H-MP), 34
Hyoid myotomy, 176
Hypoglossal nerve, 9
Hypoglossal nerve stimulation (HGNS)
  hypoglossal nerve stimulation, 80
  Imthera® system, 81
Hypoglossal/lingual artery neurovascular bundle (HLNVB), 67
Hypoxia, 140

I
ICA. *See* Internal carotid artery (ICA)
ICAp. *See* Internal carotid artery (ICAp)
ICSD-3. *See* International Classification Systems of Disorders version 3 (ICSD-3)
i-gel®, 113
Imaging
  cephalometry, 34–35
  CT, 35–37
  MRI, 37–38
  OSA, 33
Insulated coagulation-suction tube, 123
Internal carotid artery (ICA), 95
  anatomy, 98
  surgical considerations, 98
International Classification Systems of Disorders version 3 (ICSD-3), 167
Intubation, 140

J
Jennings® (Piling), 87

L
Laryngopharyngeal reflux, 222
Lateral pharyngeal wall, 93–99
Lingual nerve (LN), 99, 102
Lingual Neurovascular Bundle, 205
Lingual tonsil hypertrophy, 222
Lingual tonsils, 9

M
MAD. *See* Mandibular advancement device (MAD)
Magnetic resonance angiography (MRA), 38
Magnetic resonance imaging (MRI)
  lingual artery, 38
  lymphoid tissue and muscle, 37
Malis Bipolar® (Codman), 123
Mandibular advancement device (MAD), 34
Maryland dissector, 88, 89
Maxillo-mandibular advancement (MMA), 34, 79
MedRobotics-Flex System®, 191, 194, 218
Midazolam®, 42
Middle East
  HMC, 198
  Mallampati–Friedman scores, 201
  obesity, 197, 198
  overweight, 197, 198
  postoperative management, 201
  preoperative evaluation, 199–200
  QRSC, 199
MMA. *See* Maxillo-mandibular advancement (MMA)
Modified Cormack–Lehane view, 56
Monopolar cautery, 122, 218, 219, 223
MRA. *See* Magnetic resonance angiography (MRA)
Multilevel surgery
  BRP, 74
  ESP, 73
  retropalatal and retrolingual obstruction, 71
  UPPP, 72

N
Nasotracheal intubation, 189
Nausea management, 140–141
NOHL classification system, 169

O
Obesity, 197
Obstructive sleep apnea (OSA), 1, 114–115, 204
  airway management, 110, 112, 113
  anatomic characteristics, 13
  anatomical phenotypes, 14
  BMI, 17
  cardiovascular stimulation, 109
  cephalogram, 16
  fiber-optic endoscopy, 14
  Friedman's tongue palate classification, 15
  functional phenotypes, 14
  intraoperative management, 114
  lingual tonsil hypertrophy, 17
  Mallampati score, 18
  micro/retrognathia phenotypes, 18
  noncardiac surgery, 109

Obstructive sleep apnea (OSA) (*cont.*)
  pharyngeal airway, 16
  physical examination, 14
  postoperative care management
    analgesia, 114–115
    CPAP, 115
    oxygenation, 115
  preoperative evaluation, 110
  REM, 109
  tonsillectomy, 16
  tracheostomy, 117–118
  Woodson's classification, 16
Obstructive sleep apnea hypopnea syndrome (OSAHS), 143
  BMI, 56–57
  cardiopulmonary and neurologic sequela, 51
  DISE, 57
  dysphagia, 53
  Friedman staging system, 55–56
  laryngeal and hypopharyngeal exposure, 54
  lingual tonsil, 56
  malignant neoplasms, 55
  Modified Cormack–Lehane view, 56
  nasal deformity, 54
  phenol–glycerol technique, 55
  preoperative and perioperative management, 52
  PSG, 52–53
  surgery, 203
Obstructive sleep apnea syndrome (OSAS), 21, 184
Oral appliance therapy, 11, 170
Oropharynx, 93–102
  PPS (*see* Parapharyngeal space (PPS))
  transoral robotic surgery, 91, 92
Orotracheal/nasotracheal intubation, 140
OSA Program in Singapore and India, 205–207
OSAHS. *See* Obstructive sleep apnea/hypopnea syndrome (OSAHS)

P
Pain management, 140–141
Palatine tonsil, 93–99
Palatopharyngeal reconstructive surgery, 206
Pang–Woodson technique, 73
Parapharyngeal space (PPS)
  blood supply, 96–99
  BOT, 99–102
  glossopharyngeal nerve, 99
  LN, 99
PAS. *See* Posterior airway space (PAS)
PDT. *See* Percutaneous dilation tracheostomy (PDT)
Percutaneous dilation tracheostomy (PDT), 117
Phenotype
  anatomical, 14
  functional, 14
  micro/retrognathia, 18
  psychological, 14, 18–20
Phenotypization, 218
Polysomnography (PSG), 22
  AHI, 52
  ambulatory sleep testing, 29
  treatments, 53
POSA. *See* Positional OSA (POSA)
Positional OSA (POSA), 168, 169
Positional therapy, 171
Posterior airway space (PAS), 124
Propofol®, 42, 43, 45, 46
PSG. *See* Polysomnography (PSG)
Psychological phenotype, 14, 18–20

Q
Qatar foundation, 198–199
Qatar Robotic Surgery Center (QRSC), 199
QRSC. *See* Qatar Robotic Surgery Center (QRSC)

R
Radiofrequency base-of-tongue reduction (RFBOT), 78
Rapid eye movement (REM), 109
REM. *See* Rapid eye movement (REM)
RERA. *See* Respiratory Event Related Arousal (RERA)
Respiratory Event Related Arousal (RERA), 26
Respiratory inductive plethysmography (RIP), 26
Revision surgery, 171
RFBOT. *See* Radiofrequency base-of-tongue reduction (RFBOT)
RIP. *See* Respiratory inductive plethysmography (RIP)
Robotic surgery technology, 185
Robotic system
  cannula, 88
  Crowe-Davis® mouth gag, 87, 88
  da Vinci® Surgical System, 84
  Davis-Meyer® blades (Karl Storz), 87, 88
  Dedo®, 85, 86
  docking, 87–89
  FK-WO® retractor, 87
  Goettingen® retractor, 88
  Goettingen® table, 85, 86
  instrument table, 89

maxillary and mandibular dentition, 85, 86
nasotracheal/orotracheal intubation, 85
operating room configuration, 84, 85
sterile drape, 87
surgeon's console, 84
3-D high-definition camera, 87
TORS, 83
vision cart, 85
Xi system, 84
Royal Adelaide Experience, 210–211
Royal Adelaide Hospital, 210

S

SADs. *See* Supraglottic airway devices (SADs)
Safety
ASA classification system, 145
complication rates, 145
dysphagia and odynophagia, 146
glossectomy and uvulopalatopharyngoplasty, 145
novel procedure, 144
short and long-term swallowing, 146
Salvage surgery, 221–222
SCOPER categorization system, 23, 24
SDB. *See* Sleep-disordered breathing (SDB)
SGM. *See* Styloglossus muscle (SGM)
SJMHS. *See* St. Joseph Mercy health system (SJMHS)
SLA. *See* Superior laryngeal artery (SLA)
Sleep apnea, 160, 162
Sleep endoscopy, 41, 42
Sleep surgery community, 2
Sleep-disordered breathing (SDB), 44
Sleep-related breathing disorders (SBD)
AHI, 21
ambulatory monitoring devices, 30
ambulatory sleep testing, 29, 30
body position and limb movements recording, 28
cardiovascular parameters recording, 28
classification, 22–23
gas exchange assessment, 27
hypopnea, 23
macro–micro structural analysis, 25–26
OSAS, 21
polysomnographic report, 28–29
RERA, 26
respiratory effort, 26
SCOPER categorization system, 23, 24
snoring recording, 27
SMILE. *See* Submucosal minimally invasive lingual excision (SMILE)
Sphincter pharyngoplasty technique, 73
SPM. *See* Stylopharyngeus muscle (SPM)
ST. *See* Surgical tracheostomy (ST)
St. Joseph Mercy health system (SJMHS), 176, 177
Styloglossus (SG), 9
Styloglossus muscle (SGM), 93
Stylopharyngeus muscle (SPM)
fascial system (styloid diaphragm), 93
Submucosal minimally invasive lingual excision (SMILE), 78
Superior laryngeal artery (SLA), 105, 106
Supraglottic airway devices (SADs), 112, 113
Supraglottic larynx
aryepiglottic fold, 102
blood supply, 105–106
bucco-pharyngeal gap, 104
dorsal lingual arteries, 105
hyoid bone, 103
pharyngeal tongue, 103
surgical considerations, 105
vestibular folds, 102
Supraglottoplasty
laryngeal vessels, 130–132
supra-hyoid epiglottis, 130
tracheostomy, 132–134
"V-shape" epiglottoplasty, 130
Surgical tracheostomy (ST), 117
Swallowing, 159–164

T

Target-controlled infusion (TCI), 178, 181
TBR. *See* Tongue base reduction (TBR)
TCI. *See* Target-controlled infusion (TCI)
Thornton snoring scale, 148
3-D high-definition camera, 87
Three-dimensional multidetector computed tomography (3D MDCT), 35
3D MDCT. *See* Three-dimensional multidetector computed tomography (3D MDCT)
Thyrohoidpexy, 176
TLM. *See* Trans-oral laser microsurgery (TLM)
TLS. *See* Trans-oral laser surgery (TLS)
Tongue base, 160, 161, 163
Tongue base reduction (TBR), 188
hypoglossal nerve, 129
left-sided lingual tonsillectomy, 127–128
lingual arteries, 129
PAS, 124
residual obstruction evaluation, 128–129
right-side lingual tonsillectomy, 124–126
3D HD da Vinci® camera, 129, 130

Tongue base reduction with Hyoid-Epiglottoplasty (TBRHE), 1
Tongue body displacement, 122
Tongue pathophysiology
  characteristics, 10
  GG, 9
  human Tongue, anatomy, 8–9
  hypoglossal nerve, 9
  intrinsic muscles, 8
  lingual tonsils, 9
  musculature, 8
  REM sleep, 10
  transverse muscle, 9
Tracheostomy
  PDT, 117
  Seldinger technique, 117
  ST, 117
Trans-oral laser microsurgery (TLM), 191, 192
Trans-oral laser surgery (TLS), 193
Trans-oral robotic surgery (TORS), 83, 101, 102, 105, 206
  approach, 124
  DISE, 64, 65, 177, 178
  epiglottic prolapse, 195
  epiglottidopexy, 180
  hyoid epiglottopexy, 187
  hypopharyngeal obstruction, 180
  laryngoscopy, 180
  mandibular advancement treatments, 191
  MedRobotics-Flex-System, 191
  nasogastric tube insertion, 188
  nasotracheal intubation, 189
  oropharyngeal and supraglottic neoplasm, 64
  oropharynx, 190
  OSA, 179
  OSAHS, 67
  peri-operative management, 189
  pharyngoplasty/septoplasty, 192
  postoperative Care, 66
  robot block time, 178
  SJMHS, 177
  snoring and sleep apnea, 181
  surgical technique, 65–66
  TCI, 181
  TLM, 191
  TLS, 193
  tongue base hypertrophy, 195
  tongue base/retrolingual region, 180
  tracheostomy, 117, 188, 190, 193 (*see* Transoral robotic surgical (TORS))
  urological and gynecological procedures, 190

U

Upper airways (UAW), 9
UPPP. *See* Uvulopalatopharyngoplasty (UPPP)
Uvulopalatopharyngoplasty (UPPP), 63, 64, 71–73, 184

V

Vicini–Montevecchi technique, 73
Vision cart, 83–85
VOTE classification system, 169

W

Weight loss, 170

X

Xi system, 84

Printed by Printforce, the Netherlands